THE AGELESS MIND

MEDITATION'S SECRET PATH TO YOUTHFUL LIVING

AMBROSE HINES

Copyright © 2023 by Ambrose Hines

All rights reserved. No part of this book may be used or reproduced in any form whatsoever without written permission except in the case of brief quotations in critical articles or reviews.

For more information, or to book an event, contact:

ambrose@ambrosehines.com

www.ambrosehines.com

(f) Ambrose Hines

(⊙) Ambrose Hines

Cover design by Lisa Immelman / Ambrose Hines

First Edition: December 2023

THE AGELESS MIND

ABOUT THE AUTHOR

In *The Ageless Mind*, Ambrose Hines delves into the profound impact of meditative practices on the journey to eternal youth. Drawing from a decade-long immersion in Transcendental Meditation, the narrative is woven with the threads of diverse experiences garnered across the United States, Europe, and Africa.

Ambrose Hines's journey, shaped by a background in finance and business, includes an MBA from the esteemed Kellogg School of Management and a Master's degree from The Johns Hopkins University. The unique lens provided by a career in investment banking and corporate finance consulting adds a distinctive layer to the narrative. Through this lens, the author shares insights into the challenges of sustaining mental and physical well-being in the face of the relentless pressures of contemporary life.

The author was raised in Atlanta, Georgia, but currently resides in South Africa. The author is currently an entrepreneur that spends his spare time working with the youth as well as meditating with different groups around the world.

THE AGELESS MIND

PREFACE

In the pages of this book, readers are not presented with a mere compilation of meditative practices but, instead, offered a living testament to the profound influence of meditation on the intricate facets of aging, stress reduction, and holistic well-being. This literary journey serves as a bridge, gracefully connecting the timeless art of meditation with the relentless pace of modern existence.

This book is more than a guide; it is a narrative that articulates the deep-seated impact of meditation on the various dimensions of life, inviting readers to explore the harmonious convergence between inner peace and the unyielding demands of contemporary living. It stands as a testament to the belief that tranquility and longevity are not elusive aspirations reserved for serene retreats but are, indeed, within reach for everyone, even amidst the whirlwind of hectic schedules and demanding careers.

Through insightful anecdotes drawn from personal experiences, the author sheds light on the path to ageless living. The book seamlessly weaves together the ancient wisdom of meditation with practical insights tailored for today's challenges, making a compelling case for the integration of mindfulness into the very fabric of our daily lives.

THE AGELESS MIND

"*The Ageless Mind* is a transformative journey that rejuvenates the soul and mind. Since I started following its meditation techniques, I feel more vibrant and youthful. It's not just a book; it's a fountain of youth!"

-Emily R.

"This book has been a revelation. The unique meditation practices described in *The Ageless Mind* have significantly improved my mental clarity and reduced stress. I've never felt more alive and connected to my younger self."

-Michael T

"As someone who has always been skeptical about meditation, this was a game-changer. The simplicity and effectiveness of the methods have not only made me a believer but also visibly rejuvenated my spirit and body."

-Sarah J.

THE AGELESS MIND

CONTENTS

Chapter 1: Laying the Foundations — 01

Chapter 2: An Anti-Aging Tool — 13

Chapter 3: Better Sleep — 25

Chapter 4: The Fountain of Youth — 39

Chapter 5: Brain Health — 49

Chapter 6: Body and Mind — 75

Chapter 7: Daily Integration — 89

Chapter 8: The Art of Mindful Eating — 105

Chapter 9: Movement as Medicine — 129

Final Reflection: — 157

References: — 161

THE AGELESS MIND

CHAPTER 1
LAYING THE FOUNDATIONS: UNDERSTANDING HOW MEDITATION AFFECTS AGING

INTRODUCTION

Meditation is a timeless practice that has transcended boundaries and epochs, earning its place in the realm of ageless wisdom. Originating from the serene monasteries of the East to the bustling cities of the modern world, meditation has evolved into a universal quest for inner peace and self-discovery. It is more than just a spiritual journey; it is a gateway to rejuvenating the mind and body, offering a path to a more youthful and vibrant life.

As we embark on this enlightening journey, our focus will be to understand meditation in its essence - its various forms, its rich history, and most importantly, its profound influence on the aging process. This chapter aims to build a foundational understanding, demystifying the science behind meditation and how it emerges as a potent tool in countering aging.

AGING

Aging is a natural process that occurs in all living organisms as they get older. It is the gradual decline in the body's ability to repair and regenerate cells, which results in physical changes such as wrinkles, gray hair, and decreased mobility, as well as mental changes such as memory loss and decreased cognitive function.

As we age, our bodies go through a number of physical changes. Our skin becomes thinner and less elastic, which makes it more susceptible to damage and wrinkles. Our muscles and bones also become weaker, which can lead to a loss of mobility and balance. Additionally, our internal organs, such as the heart and lungs, may not function as efficiently as they once did.

Mental changes are also common with aging. Many people experience a decline in cognitive function, such as memory loss and difficulty with problem-solving and decision-making. However, it's important to note that these changes are not universal and can vary greatly among individuals.

While genetics play a significant role in aging, environmental factors such as diet, exercise, and exposure to toxins can also impact the aging process. For example, a diet high in processed foods and sugar can accelerate the aging of cells, while regular exercise can help maintain muscle mass and cognitive function.

THE ANCIENT ROOTS OF MEDITATION

Meditation has a rich history that spans across cultures and civilizations. In the ancient Vedas of India, meditation was used as a means of spiritual enlightenment and a way to connect with the divine. In Japan, Zen meditation was focused on achieving inner peace and balance. Similarly, in Chinese Taoism, meditation was used as a tool to develop one's

Qi or vital energy.

Despite the different origins, what unites these practices is their aim to cultivate a state of deep inner calm and clarity. Meditation has been a constant companion to humanity in its quest for understanding and tranquility. It has been practiced by sages, ascetics, and common people alike, and has been passed down through generations across the globe.

By tracing the historical journey of meditation, we can gain a deeper appreciation of its transformative power. The roots of meditation lie in ancient wisdom, and its influence continues to be felt today as people from all walks of life turn to meditation as a way to find inner peace and balance amidst the challenges of modern life.

SCIENTIFIC PERSPECTIVE ON MEDITATION AND AGING

Meditation has become increasingly popular among people of all ages, and research has shown that it can have significant benefits for aging individuals. From a scientific perspective, meditation has been found to have positive effects on both physical and mental health, which are key factors in the process of aging.

The intersection of meditation and modern science has unveiled fascinating insights into how this practice influences the aging process. Studies reveal that regular meditation contributes to physiological changes at the cellular level, notably in the lengthening of telomeres, key indicators of cellular aging. Such findings provide compelling evidence of meditation's role in promoting longevity.

In addition to cellular benefits, meditation has shown promising effects on cognitive functions, enhancing memory and focus, often impacted by the aging process. Groundbreaking studies and research have begun to unravel the physiological and cognitive benefits of meditation, offering a new perspective on how we can approach aging healthily and mindfully.

CELLULAR BENEFITS OF MEDITATION

Meditation has been found to have numerous cellular benefits, which are particularly important for aging individuals. Studies have shown that regular meditation practice can help to reduce cellular aging, increase telomerase activity, improve mitochondrial function, and reduce inflammation in the body. These cellular benefits can contribute to overall health and well-being, helping individuals to age more gracefully and maintain their physical and cognitive abilities for longer.

IMPACT ON TELOMERES

One of the most significant findings in the study of meditation and aging is its effect on telomeres. Telomeres are the protective caps at the ends of our chromosomes, and their length is a key indicator of cellular aging and overall health. Research indicates that regular meditation can help maintain telomere length, effectively slowing the cellular aging process. This is attributed to the reduction of stress hormones and oxidative stress, both of which are known to contribute to telomere shortening.

REDUCTION OF INFLAMMATORY RESPONSES

Chronic inflammation is a known contributor to aging and various age-related diseases. Meditation has been shown to downregulate genes responsible for inflammatory reactions, thereby reducing the body's inflammatory response. This not only impacts aging but also improves overall health and reduces the risk of numerous inflammation-related conditions.

COGNITIVE BENEFITS OF MEDITATION

Cognition refers to the mental processes involved in acquiring, processing, and using information. It encompasses a range of abilities, such as perception, attention, memory, language, and problem-solving. Cognition enables us to make sense of the world around us, to understand and retain information, and to engage in complex decision-making and problem-solving tasks. Therefore, cognitive abilities are crucial for our daily functioning and overall well-being.

ENHANCING MEMORY AND FOCUS

As we age, cognitive functions such as memory and focus can decline. Meditation, however, has shown promise in enhancing these cognitive abilities. Studies have demonstrated that regular meditation practice leads to changes in brain regions associated with memory, attention, and executive functions. This is particularly significant in the context of age-related cognitive decline.

NEUROPLASTICITY AND BRAIN AGING

Neuroplasticity refers to the brain's ability to reorganize itself by forming new neural connections throughout life. Meditation has been found to promote neuroplasticity, which is crucial in mitigating the effects of brain aging. By fostering a healthier brain environment, meditation can aid in maintaining cognitive functions and mental agility in older adults.

MENTAL HEALTH AND EMOTIONAL WELL-BEING

Beyond cognitive enhancement, meditation contributes significantly to mental health and emotional well-being. Practices like mindfulness meditation have been linked to lower rates of depression, anxiety, and mood-related disorders among older adults. The calming effect of meditation can lead to a more positive outlook on life, increased emotional resilience, and a better quality of life.

MEDITATION AS A STRESS-RELIEF TOOL

Meditation is a powerful tool for stress relief, and this benefit becomes particularly valuable as we age. High stress levels can have detrimental effects on both cognitive and physical health. Through various meditation techniques, individuals can learn to manage stress, reduce the body's production of stress hormones, and promote a sense of calm. This aspect of meditation is crucial in enhancing overall well-being and resilience in the face of life's challenges.

SOCIAL CONNECTION AND COMMUNITY BUILDING

Engaging in meditation with different groups around the world not only offers personal benefits but also fosters a sense of social connection and community. As older adults, maintaining an active social life and a sense of belonging is essential for mental and emotional well-being. Meditation groups provide an opportunity to connect with like-minded individuals, share experiences, and build a supportive community. This sense of belonging can contribute to a more fulfilling and enriching life in one's later years.

LONGEVITY AND OVERALL WELL-BEING

The convergence of these benefits – from maintaining cellular health to enhancing cognitive function and emotional well-being – suggests that meditation is more than a tool for stress relief; it is a powerful practice for promoting longevity and a healthier, more youthful existence. By integrating meditation into daily life, individuals of all ages can tap into its age-defying benefits, leading to not just a longer life, but a richer and more fulfilling one.

Practical Tips:
Starting Your Meditation Journey

For those new to meditation, the journey begins with small, yet significant steps. This part of the chapter will offer practical advice and simple techniques for beginners. Emphasizing the importance of starting with manageable goals, we will explore basic breathing exercises, mindfulness practices, and guided visualizations. These methods serve as accessible entry points into the broader world of meditation, paving the way for a deeper and more impactful practice.

SETTING THE STAGE FOR MEDITATION

- **CREATE A QUIET SPACE**
  Choose a peaceful spot in your home where you won't be disturbed. It could be a corner of a room, a spot by a window, or even a peaceful outdoor area. The environment should feel serene and inviting.

- **COMFORTABLE SEATING** Sit on a cushion, chair, or mat, ensuring your back is straight yet relaxed. Comfort is crucial, as physical discomfort can distract from the meditation experience.

- **SCHEDULE REGULAR TIMES**
  Consistency is key. Try to meditate at the same time every day, whether it's in the morning to start your day with clarity or in the evening to unwind.

BASIC BREATHING EXERCISES

- **MINDFUL BREATHING**
  Sit quietly and focus on your natural breathing pattern. Notice the sensation of air entering and leaving your nostrils, or the rise and

fall of your chest. Whenever your mind wanders, gently bring your focus back to your breath.

- **COUNTED BREATHS**
  Breathe in slowly while counting to four, hold your breath for a count of four, then exhale for a count of four. This technique helps maintain focus and deepens your breathing.

MINDFULNESS PRACTICES

- **Body Scan Meditation**
  Begin at the top of your head and slowly bring your attention down through your body, noticing any sensations, tension, or relaxation. This practice helps develop a mindful awareness of your bodily sensations.

- **Mindful Observation**
  Choose an object — a flower, a candle flame, or even a piece of fruit. Focus all your attention on this object, observing every detail about it. This practice helps train your mind to focus and be present.

GUIDED VISUALIZATIONS

Guided visualizations are a type of meditation technique that involves the use of mental imagery to promote relaxation, enhance creativity, and achieve specific goals. During a guided visualization, a person is led through a series of mental images and instructions, often accompanied by calming music or sounds, to help them imagine a specific scenario or outcome.

GUIDED IMAGERY

Use guided meditation apps or recordings where a narrator leads you through a peaceful scene or story. These can be particularly helpful for beginners who find it challenging to focus or quiet the mind.

Explore meditation apps like Headspace, Calm, Insight Timer, Breethe, Smiling Mind, Aura, and Simple Habit to access guided imagery and visualization sessions.

These apps offer a diverse range of guided meditations designed to enhance relaxation, reduce stress, and foster a peaceful state of mind.

VISUALIZING PEACEFUL SCENERY

Take a moment to close your eyes and imagine a place that brings you peace and serenity. Let your mind wander and explore the details of this place. Maybe it's a secluded beach with crystal clear water and soft white sand, or a quiet forest with towering trees and a gentle breeze. Perhaps it's a cozy room filled with warm light and comfortable furniture. Engage all your senses - what do you see, hear, and feel in this place? Take in the colors, the sounds, the textures, and the scents. Let this image fill you with a sense of calm and tranquility.

Embracing Patience And Persistence

It's important to remember that developing meditation skills takes time and patience. Don't get discouraged if you find your mind wandering during meditation - this is completely normal. Acknowledge the distraction and gently refocus on your technique.

With consistent practice, you'll find your sessions becoming deeper and more fulfilling. Stick with it, and you'll soon embrace the benefits of patience and persistence in your meditation practice.

Case Study 1:
Transformation Through Meditation

John's meditation journey began with simple steps. He started with just five minutes a day, focusing on his breath and trying to clear his mind of the relentless stream of thoughts.

The first few sessions were challenging, as he struggled to find focus, but he persisted. Gradually, these short sessions of mindfulness started to make a difference. John noticed he was feeling calmer, and his sleep quality began to improve.

Encouraged by these initial changes, John expanded his practice. He explored different meditation techniques, including guided imagery and mindfulness meditation. He began attending a local meditation group, which not only enhanced his practice but also connected him with a community of like-minded individuals.

After six months of consistent practice, the changes in John were remarkable. He reported feeling more energetic, his concentration improved, and he felt an overall sense of well-being that he hadn't experienced in years.

His family and friends noticed the change too; John seemed more present, more engaged, and noticeably more content.

Perhaps the most significant change was observed in John's approach to life's challenges. Situations that would have previously caused him stress now seemed more manageable. He found himself responding to challenges with a calmness and clarity that was new to him.

John's journey with meditation was transformative. It not only improved his physical and mental health but also offered him a new perspective on life. At 60, John felt rejuvenated, proving that it's never too late to embrace the practice of meditation and experience its life-altering benefits.

Conclusion For Chapter 1
Forming The Cornerstone

In this opening chapter, we've laid the groundwork for understanding the profound impact of meditation on the aging process. We embarked on a journey through the history of meditation, tracing its roots across various cultures and its evolution into a tool for modern wellness.

Additionally, we explored the scientific aspects, discussing how meditation can positively affect cellular aging and improve cognitive function, among other benefits. This provided a tangible understanding of meditation's role in promoting a healthier, more youthful life.

Chapter Key Points

1. Meditation's historical roots span diverse cultures, evolving into a modern wellness practice.

2. Scientific research supports meditation's positive effects on cellular aging and cognitive function.

3. Practical tips offered a starting point for beginners, highlighting simple techniques to ease into the practice of meditation. These methods serve as a foundation for developing a deeper, more enriching meditation experience.

4. John's case study exemplified the transformative power of meditation. His journey from stress and fatigue to a state of

renewed energy and clarity was a testament to the positive changes meditation can bring about at any age.

SUMMARY AND PREPARATION FOR CHAPTER 2

As we close this chapter, we hope to have ignited a sense of curiosity and motivation to explore meditation further. In the next chapter, we will delve deeper into how meditation aids in stress reduction and its implications for the aging process, continuing our journey towards understanding how this timeless practice can lead to a life of wellness and vitality.

Chapter 2
An Anti-Aging Tool: Meditation For Stress Reduction

Introduction

Stress is a significant player in the intricate dance of life, often lurking in the background but exerting a profound impact. In today's fast-paced world, stress has become more than just a fleeting emotional state. It has become a constant presence, subtly weaving its way into our daily lives. The consequences of chronic stress are far-reaching, especially in how it accelerates the aging process. It's important to recognize and manage stress effectively to prevent it from taking a toll on our overall wellbeing.

Chronic stress, often dismissed as an unavoidable aspect of modern life, is more than just a psychological burden; it is a critical factor that influences our biological systems and contributes significantly to premature aging. This chapter aims to delve deep into the complex relationship between stress and aging, shedding light on how this invisible adversary affects our cellular health, brain function, and overall vitality.

From the hurried steps of our morning routines to the unending demands of our professional lives, stress is omnipresent. Its implications, however, extend far beyond the immediate feeling of being overwhelmed. Chronic stress sets off a cascade of biochemical reactions in our bodies, which, over time, wear down our physiological resilience, leading to accelerated aging and a host of age-related diseases.

The Science Of Stress And Aging

Stress and aging are two intertwined phenomena that have been the subject of extensive scientific inquiry. The impact of stress on aging can be seen at various physiological levels, including DNA damage, inflammation, and telomere shortening. Over time, these effects can accelerate the aging process and increase the risk of age-related diseases such as Alzheimer's, cardiovascular disease, and cancer. Recent research has shed light on the intricate mechanisms through which stress contributes to aging, including the role of stress hormones and oxidative stress. Understanding these mechanisms can help us develop effective strategies to mitigate the negative impact of stress on our health and wellbeing.

THE ROLE OF CORTISOL

Cortisol, often termed the 'stress hormone,' is central to our body's response to stress. It's essential for survival, orchestrating the 'fight or flight' response in threatening situations. However, the modern lifestyle has led to prolonged exposure to elevated cortisol levels, which can be detrimental to our health.

Chronic high cortisol levels have been linked to a multitude of health issues. They can lead to hypertension, increase the risk of heart disease, and weaken immune function.

The detrimental effects of cortisol also extend to our mental health, contributing to conditions like anxiety and depression. This section will examine how sustained high cortisol levels impact various body systems, accelerating the aging process.

OXIDATIVE STRESS AND CELLULAR AGING

Another key player in the stress-aging dynamic is oxidative stress. This occurs when there's an imbalance between free radicals and antioxidants in the body. Free radicals are unstable molecules that can damage cells, leading to cellular aging.

Stress-induced oxidative stress is particularly harmful as it accelerates the wear and tear on cells, contributing to the aging process at a cellular level. Antioxidants play a crucial role in neutralizing free radicals, thus mitigating the effects of oxidative stress. The discussion will explore how stress contributes to oxidative stress and the importance of antioxidants in countering this effect.

BRAIN AGING AND NEUROTRANSMITTERS

Chronic stress also exerts a profound impact on the brain. It affects neurotransmitter systems, alters brain structure, and can lead to cognitive decline. This part of the chapter will delve into how stress hormones affect neurotransmitters like serotonin and dopamine, which are crucial for mood regulation and cognitive function.

MEDITATION **A**S **A** **S**TRESS **R**EDUCER

In the quest to mitigate the effects of stress and its aging implications, meditation emerges as a powerful and accessible tool. This ancient practice, with its myriad forms and techniques, offers a pathway to tranquility and resilience against life's inevitable stressors.

Here, we delve deeper into three key meditation techniques – Mindfulness Meditation, Focused Attention Meditation, and Loving-Kindness Meditation – each uniquely effective in combating stress.

DEEP-DIVE INTO MINDFULNESS MEDITATION

At the heart of mindfulness meditation is the art of cultivating awareness and presence. This practice involves a conscious attention to the present moment, observing thoughts, feelings, and sensations without judgment or attachment.

UNDERSTANDING MINDFULNESS

Mindfulness is about being fully engaged with the here and now. It's not about emptying the mind, but rather acknowledging and accepting whatever arises in one's consciousness.

TECHNIQUES FOR CULTIVATING AWARENESS

BREATH AWARENESS

Begin by focusing on your breath – its rhythm, the sensation of air moving in and out of your lungs. Each time your mind wanders, gently bring your attention back to your breath.

BODY SCAN

Progressively move your focus through different parts of your body, from the tips of your toes to the top of your head. Observe any tension or sensations you feel in each area.

MINDFUL OBSERVATION

Select an object and focus all your attention on it. Notice its color, shape, texture, and other qualities, fully engaging with the present moment.

FOCUSED ATTENTION MEDITATION

Focused attention meditation hones the mind's ability to concentrate on a single point, thought, or object, which helps in breaking the cycle of stress-induced thought patterns.

BREATHING MEDITATION

Choose a quiet place and sit comfortably. Focus solely on your breath, following each inhalation and exhalation. When your mind wanders, gently redirect it back to your breathing.

MANTRA MEDITATION

Select a word, phrase, or sound as your mantra. Repeat it silently, allowing the repetition to anchor your mind. This practice helps to clear the mind of scattered thoughts and brings about a sense of inner peace.

STEP-BY-STEP GUIDE FOR BEGINNERS

1. **Find a Comfortable Position:** Sit in a relaxed but alert position, maintaining good posture.

2. **Select Your Focus:** Choose your breath or a mantra as your point of focus.

3. **Set a Timer:** Begin with short periods, like 5 to 10 minutes, and gradually increase your practice time.

4. **Gently Return to Focus**: Each time your mind wanders, acknowledge it without judgment and return to your chosen focus.

LOVING-KINDNESS MEDITATION (METTA)

Loving-Kindness Meditation, also known as Metta in Pali, is a powerful practice for cultivating compassion and empathy towards oneself and others. It involves repeating phrases that express heartfelt wishes for happiness, peace, and well-being. By focusing on positive emotions and intentions, this practice can help reduce stress, anxiety, and negative thinking patterns, and promote feelings of joy, love, and connection.

PHRASES USED IN METTA MEDITATION

Common phrases include "May I be happy," "May I be healthy," "May I be safe," and "May I live with ease." After directing these phrases to yourself, extend them to others – loved ones, acquaintances, and even those you may have conflicts with.

BENEFITS OF LOVING-KINDNESS MEDITATION

- **FOSTERS EMOTIONAL RESILIENCE**
  Regular practice can increase positive emotions and decrease negative ones, leading to greater emotional stability.

- **ENHANCES SOCIAL CONNECTEDNESS**
  By nurturing feelings of kindness and compassion, Metta meditation can improve relationships and foster a sense of connectedness with others.

- **REDUCES STRESS-RELATED SYMPTOMS**
  This form of meditation can decrease symptoms of stress, anxiety, and depression, promoting an overall sense of well-being.

Practical Tips To Reduce Stress Through Meditation

To effectively reduce stress through meditation, it's important to incorporate it into daily life. Here are some practical tips:

START SMALL

Begin with short sessions, even just 5-10 minutes daily, and gradually increase the duration.

REGULAR PRACTICE

Consistency is key. Try to meditate at the same time each day to establish a routine.

CREATE A CALMING ENVIRONMENT

Choose a quiet, comfortable spot for meditation. You may use soothing music or aromatherapy to enhance the experience.

MINDFUL ACTIVITIES

Incorporate mindfulness into everyday activities like walking or eating. This helps in staying grounded in the present moment, reducing stress.

Case Study 2: Overcoming Stress Through Meditation

Jean, a 45-year-old marketing executive, faced a high-stress life that left her overwhelmed and anxious. Frequent headaches and sleep disturbances were her constant companions. She reluctantly turned to meditation as a last resort.

Sarah's journey began with guided mindfulness meditation using a mobile app. Initially skeptical, she committed to short daily sessions.

The first few weeks were challenging; her mind wandered incessantly, and she struggled to find a quiet moment amidst her busy schedule. Yet, she persevered.

Gradually, she began to notice subtle changes. Her sleep quality improved, and the headaches became less frequent. She felt more composed in dealing with daily stressors. Meditation slowly transformed from a task into a sanctuary—a time to disconnect from external chaos and reconnect with her inner peace.

Encouraged by these improvements, Sarah explored other meditation forms. She tried focused attention meditation, finding solace in its simplicity. The act of focusing solely on her breath or a chosen mantra helped declutter her mind, bringing a sense of clarity she hadn't felt in years.

Curious about the broader implications of meditation, Sarah ventured into loving-kindness meditation. This practice, initially foreign to her, allowed her to cultivate feelings of compassion not just towards herself but also towards her colleagues, friends, and even the strangers she encountered daily. This expansion of empathy had a surprising effect—her relationships began to improve, conflicts seemed less daunting, and she felt a deeper connection with those around her.

Sarah's commitment to meditation extended beyond her individual practice. She initiated a meditation group at her workplace. This small community of like-minded individuals met weekly, sharing experiences and supporting each other in their stress-reduction journey. The group became a source of motivation and accountability, helping her maintain consistency in her practice.

Over months, the benefits of meditation became more pronounced. Sarah's anxiety levels dropped significantly. She found herself more present and engaged in her interactions, her creativity at work flourished, and her overall mood improved. The physical manifestations of stress, like headaches and sleep issues, were now rare occurrences.

Her journey didn't just alleviate her stress; it redefined her approach to life. She became more resilient, patient, and joyful. Meditation's impact extended beyond her personal well-being; it influenced her professional performance and relationships, demonstrating the profound, far-reaching effects of a consistent meditation practice.

Conclusion For Chapter 2: Meditation's Ageless Gift

In Chapter 2, "An Anti-Aging Tool: Meditation for Stress Reduction," we've explored the profound role of meditation in alleviating stress and its transformative effects on the aging process. Through the lens of scientific research and personal anecdotes, we've witnessed how meditation serves as a powerful tool for mitigating the detrimental impact of stress on both mind and body.

We've uncovered the intricate mechanisms through which meditation reduces stress hormones, bolsters emotional resilience, and enhances overall well-being. The story of Sarah who harnessed meditation's potential to navigate life's challenges serve as a testament to its efficacy.

As we conclude this chapter, the message is clear: meditation is not just a practice but a way of life, a path to tranquillity and vitality. In the chapters that follow, we will continue to explore the multifaceted benefits of meditation, delving deeper into its potential to rejuvenate the mind and body, ultimately leading us on the path to ageless living.

Chapter Key Points

UNDERSTANDING STRESS AND AGING

We delved into how chronic stress accelerates aging, discussing the detrimental role of cortisol, oxidative stress, and the impact on neurotransmitters. This foundation set the stage for appreciating meditation's role in combating these effects.

EXPLORING MEDITATION TECHNIQUES

We explored various meditation methods, each with unique benefits for stress reduction. Mindfulness Meditation enhances present-moment awareness, Focused Attention Meditation cultivates a calm and centered mind, and Loving-Kindness Meditation nurtures empathy and emotional resilience.

SARAH'S TRANSFORMATIVE JOURNEY

Sarah's story illustrated the practical application of these techniques. Her journey from a high-stress lifestyle to a more balanced and peaceful existence highlighted the real-world impact of meditation. Her experiences provided valuable insights into how consistent meditation practice can lead to significant improvements in stress management and overall quality of life.

PRACTICAL APPLICATION

The chapter offered practical tips for incorporating meditation into daily routines, emphasizing the importance of personalization and consistency in practice. These guidelines aim to help readers overcome common challenges and integrate meditation seamlessly into their lives.

UNDERSTANDING STRESS MANAGEMENT THROUGH MEDITATION

This chapter has provided us with a deeper understanding of how meditation is a powerful tool in managing stress, a common challenge in our daily lives.

We explored various meditation techniques and their effectiveness in reducing stress-related symptoms, contributing to a more balanced and serene lifestyle.

BROADER BENEFITS BEYOND STRESS REDUCTION

Beyond its impact on stress, meditation has been shown to have far-reaching benefits, influencing other areas of our health and wellness. This holistic approach is what makes meditation an invaluable practice in our lives.

<u>SUMMARY AND PREPARATION FOR CHAPTER 3</u>

As we draw this chapter to a close, we reflect on the intricate and diverse benefits meditation offers, particularly in the realm of stress management.

However, the journey through the world of meditation reveals many more facets, each contributing uniquely to our overall well-being.

In our upcoming chapter, we will delve into the essential relationship between meditation and sleep quality, a crucial aspect often overlooked in discussions about health and aging.

Sleep, often underestimated, is indeed a fundamental pillar of our health, playing a critical role in our vitality, especially as we age.

We will explore the profound ways in which meditation can enhance the quality of our sleep. Understanding this link is essential, as quality sleep is a major contributor to maintaining youthfulness and overall well-being.

The chapter will dive into how meditation not only aids in achieving a deeper and more restful sleep but also addresses common sleep-related issues, thus contributing to a more vibrant and youthful life.

Discover how embracing meditation can be a key element in crafting a life marked by vitality and youthfulness. We will explore practical meditation techniques, backed by scientific research and personal anecdotes, to demonstrate the significant impact that quality sleep, achieved through meditation, can have on our lives.

Chapter 3
Better Sleep:
The Gateway To Youth

Introduction

Sleep is often overlooked and undervalued in our fast-paced world, but it is an essential thread in the tapestry of life. As we age, the quality and quantity of our sleep become increasingly crucial for our overall health and wellbeing. This chapter emphasizes the active and vital role of sleep, especially in our later years. By prioritizing the significance of sleep and understanding its importance, we can improve our physical and mental health, and ultimately, our quality of life. Don't neglect the power of sleep - it's a crucial element that should be taken seriously at any age.

The relationship between sleep and aging is intricate. As we age, our sleep patterns change; we tend to sleep less and experience lighter, more fragmented sleep. This shift can affect everything from cognitive function to physical health.

Sleep is when the body engages in various repair processes, including muscle growth, tissue repair, protein synthesis, and the release of growth hormones essential for cell regeneration. The lack of quality sleep can accelerate the aging process, manifesting in reduced cognitive abilities, weakened immune response, and increased susceptibility to diseases like Alzheimer's, obesity, and diabetes.

THE ROLE OF MEDITATION IN IMPROVING SLEEP QUALITY

UNDERSTANDING THE SLEEP-MEDITATION CONNECTION

Meditation, with its profound calming effects on the mind and body, plays a crucial role in enhancing sleep quality. By inducing a state of deep relaxation, meditation can help break the cycle of restless thoughts and tension, which are common culprits of sleep disturbances.

This relaxed state aids in the transition into sleep, reducing the time it takes to fall asleep (sleep latency) and increasing the overall quality of sleep.

Meditation practices foster a heightened awareness of mental and physical states, helping to recognize and mitigate the signs of stress and anxiety that often interfere with sleep. By calming the mind and reducing rumination, meditation can effectively address the psychological barriers to restful sleep.

SCIENTIFIC INSIGHTS

Emerging research in the field of sleep medicine and neurology underscores the efficacy of meditation in improving sleep quality. Studies have shown that meditation activates the parasympathetic nervous system, which is responsible for calming the body and promoting the 'rest and digest' state. This activation is crucial for initiating the sleep process.

One notable study published in JAMA Internal Medicine found that mindfulness meditation significantly improved sleep quality in older adults with moderate sleep disturbances. Another research highlighted the effect of meditation on enhancing REM sleep and reducing the occurrence of sleep disorders.

These scientific insights provide a compelling argument for incorporating meditation into routines for those seeking to improve their sleep quality.

ANTI-AGING BENEFITS OF QUALITY SLEEP

Quality sleep is a potent elixir of youth. During sleep, the body undergoes critical restorative processes that are vital for physical and mental health.

This period of rest allows for cellular repair, memory consolidation, and the clearing of brain waste, which could potentially contribute to neurodegenerative diseases if accumulated.

Furthermore, sleep plays a pivotal role in maintaining hormonal balance, including the regulation of cortisol and insulin. Disruptions in these hormonal pathways due to poor sleep can accelerate aging and increase the risk of age-related diseases.

By improving sleep quality through meditation, we can enhance these regenerative processes, thereby slowing down the biological clock and promoting longevity.

Practical Tips:
Meditation Routines For Better Sleep

CREATING A PRE-SLEEP MEDITATION ROUTINE

Establishing a pre-sleep meditation routine can be a game-changer in achieving restorative sleep. This routine serves as a signal to the body and mind that it's time to unwind and prepare for sleep. A consistent pre-sleep meditation practice can help in developing a regular sleep pattern, making it easier to fall asleep and stay asleep.

CHOOSE A COMFORTABLE SPOT

Find a quiet, comfortable space where you can relax without interruption. This could be a cozy corner in your bedroom or any place that evokes a sense of tranquility.

SET A REGULAR TIME

Consistency is key. Try to meditate at the same time each evening to establish a rhythm your body can recognize and adapt to.

LIMIT EXPOSURE TO SCREENS

Reduce exposure to screens and bright lights at least an hour before your meditation, as they can disrupt the production of melatonin, a hormone that regulates sleep.

UNPLUG FROM TECHNOLOGY

In the digital age, it is easy to stay connected until the last minute. However, for a more effective pre-sleep routine, make it a habit to unplug from technology at least an hour before bedtime. This not only reduces exposure to stimulating content but also helps quiet the mind for meditation relaxation to your body.

Specific Meditation Techniques For Sleep

GUIDED SLEEP MEDITATION

Utilize guided meditations designed specifically for sleep, which often include soothing narratives or ambient sounds to lull the mind into a state of deep relaxation.

BODY SCAN MEDITATION

Start at the toes and gradually move your focus up through each part of the body. Consciously relax each area, releasing tension and allowing a sense of calm to permeate your entire body.

BREATH-FOCUSED MEDITATION

In bed, practice deep, slow breathing. Concentrate on the rhythm of your breath, letting each inhale and exhale gently ease you closer to sleep.

Incorporating Mindfulness Into Evening Routines

Complement your meditation practice with a mindful evening routine. Activities like reading, gentle stretching, or writing in a gratitude journal can further promote relaxation. Engage in these activities with full attention, letting go of the day's worries and stresses, and transitioning your mind toward peaceful rest.

Consider creating a soothing ambiance in your living space by dimming the lights and playing calming music. This can help create a serene atmosphere for your evening routine. Remember that your evening routine is sacred.

CASE STUDY 3:
THE TRANSFORMATIVE POWER OF SLEEP

Alex, a 45-year-old project manager, faced the all-too-common challenge of sleep disturbances. His life was a balancing act between demanding work schedules, family responsibilities, and trying to maintain a semblance of a social life. Over time, his sleep, often relegated to an afterthought, became increasingly fragmented and unrefreshing. Waking up tired, relying on caffeine to get through the day, and feeling irritable became his new normal.

Alex's struggle with sleep was not just an inconvenience; it began to take a significant toll on his health. He noticed a decline in his cognitive abilities – his concentration wavered, memory lapses were more frequent, and decision-making became a daunting task.

His mood swings started to strain his relationships, and a general sense of lethargy overshadowed his daily life.

THE ONSET OF SLEEP ISSUES

Alex's sleep problems began subtly – an occasional restless night here and there, initially dismissed as just bad days. However, these sporadic episodes gradually coalesced into a pattern of chronic sleep deprivation. He found himself lying awake in bed, his mind racing with the day's events or worrying about upcoming deadlines. The little sleep he did manage was shallow and interrupted, leaving him feeling exhausted in the mornings.

ALEX'S REALIZATION AND DECISION TO CHANGE

The turning point came during a routine check-up when his doctor expressed concern over Alex's elevated blood pressure and stress levels. It was a wake-up call for Alex. He realized that his sleep issues were not just a minor nuisance but a serious threat to his overall well-being. He began researching ways to improve his sleep and stumbled upon the potential benefits of meditation.

INCORPORATING MEDITATION INTO HIS ROUTINE

Initially skeptical, Alex decided to give meditation a try, spurred by the numerous positive studies he had read. He started with a simple guided sleep meditation, dedicating 15 minutes each night to the practice. The first few nights were challenging – his mind wandered constantly, and he felt more frustrated than relaxed.

However, Alex persisted, drawn by the moments of calm he experienced during his sessions. Gradually, he noticed a shift. His mind began to quiet down faster, and the transition from meditation to sleep became smoother.

Encouraged by these small victories, he began exploring other meditation techniques, such as mindfulness and deep breathing exercises.

THE POSITIVE CHANGES

Over the weeks, Alex's sleep quality started to improve significantly. The most noticeable change was how much quicker he fell asleep after meditating. His sleep was deeper, and the frequent awakenings that used to fragment his night's rest became rare occurrences.

The benefits of better sleep began to manifest in various aspects of his life. His concentration improved, making him more efficient at work. He found himself more patient and present with his family, leading to more harmonious interactions.

Physically, he felt more energized, and his reliance on caffeine diminished. His doctor noted a marked improvement in his blood pressure and stress levels during a follow-up visit.

LONG-TERM IMPACT

Alex's journey with meditation and improved sleep was transformative. It wasn't just about overcoming insomnia; it was about reclaiming his health and vitality. He discovered that quality sleep, facilitated by meditation, was a cornerstone of his well-being. It improved his mental clarity, emotional balance, and physical health, contributing to a more vibrant and energetic life.

DEEPENING HIS PRACTICE

As Alex's initial forays into meditation showed promising results, he felt encouraged to delve deeper. He started attending a weekly meditation class, seeking to enhance his understanding and technique.

These classes introduced him to different meditation styles, each offering unique benefits. He learned about the importance of posture, breathing techniques, and the power of mental imagery.

During these classes, Alex also discovered the value of community in his meditation journey. Sharing experiences with others, understanding their struggles and successes, gave him a sense of belonging and motivation.

He realized that his challenges were not unique, and this shared experience was instrumental in his continued practice.

BROADER LIFESTYLE CHANGES

Encouraged by the positive changes in his sleep and overall well-being, Alex began to implement broader lifestyle changes. He adjusted his evening routine to reduce exposure to blue light from screens, started eating lighter meals at night, and incorporated gentle physical activities like yoga and walking into his evenings. These changes complemented his meditation practice, further setting the stage for better sleep.

OVERCOMING SETBACKS

Alex's journey wasn't without its challenges. There were nights when despite meditating, sleep eluded him, and frustration crept in.

During these moments, he relied on the mindfulness techniques he learned, observing his thoughts and emotions without judgment, and gently steering his focus back to relaxation and breath.

He also maintained an open dialogue with his meditation instructor, gaining insights and personalized tips to navigate these hurdles. This support was crucial in helping him stay on course and not lose sight of his goals.

WITNESSING THE CUMULATIVE BENEFITS

Several months into his journey, the cumulative effects of Alex's new sleep habits and meditation practice were evident. His sleep tracker showed increased periods of deep sleep, and he woke up feeling genuinely refreshed.

His performance reviews at work noted his heightened focus and creativity. Friends and family remarked on his calmer demeanor and renewed zest for life. Alex also found that his meditation practice had unexpected benefits. He developed a better understanding of his thought patterns and emotional responses, leading to a more mindful approach to daily challenges.

This mindfulness transcended beyond his personal life, improving his interactions at work and deepening his relationships.

A RENEWED PERSPECTIVE ON AGING

One of the most profound realizations for Alex was the shift in his perspective on aging. He began to view sleep and meditation not as mere remedies for insomnia but as integral components of a healthy aging process. He understood that quality sleep, enhanced by meditation, was not just restoring his body each night but was actively contributing to his long-term health and vitality.

SHARING HIS EXPERIENCE

Inspired by his transformation, Alex became an advocate for meditation and sleep hygiene in his community. He started a small meditation group among his friends and colleagues, sharing techniques and experiences.

His story, relatable and inspiring, encouraged others to explore meditation as a tool for better sleep and overall well-being. Alex's journey from a sleep-deprived individual to someone who mastered the art of restful sleep through meditation is a testament to the power of perseverance, holistic health, and the mind-body connection.

His story illuminates the profound impact that quality sleep and mindfulness practices can have on all facets of life. It stands as an inspiring example of how embracing a holistic approach to sleep and stress management can lead not only to a healthier life but also to a deeper understanding of oneself.

Alex's transformative journey underscores a vital message: in the fast-paced rhythm of modern life, prioritizing sleep and mindfulness is not a luxury, but a necessity for a vibrant, healthy, and fulfilling existence.

Through his experiences, we learn that the path to wellness and rejuvenation is within our reach, guided by the simple yet powerful practice of meditation.

Conclusion For Chapter 3: Unlocking Youth's Sanctuary

In the quiet hush of Chapter 3, we've embarked on a voyage through the enigmatic realm of sleep—a realm where the rejuvenation of youth is whispered in the stillness of the night. Through the marriage of science and practicality, we've unveiled the profound significance of restorative slumber.

As we draw the curtain on this chapter, we carry with us the knowledge that sleep is more than a nightly ritual; it's a sacred rebirth, a realm where the body renews itself, the mind finds clarity, and the spirit is rekindled. It's in this ethereal sanctuary that the ageless secrets of life are subtly woven into our being.

Chapter Key Points

INTEGRAL ROLE OF SLEEP IN AGING

We delved into the critical importance of sleep in maintaining health and vitality, particularly as we age. The chapter highlighted how sleep acts as a regenerative process, crucial for cognitive functions, cellular health, and overall well-being.

MEDITATION'S IMPACT ON SLEEP QUALITY

We explored the sleep-meditation connection, revealing how meditation practices can significantly improve sleep quality. By calming the mind and body, meditation aids in regulating the sleep-wake cycle, reducing the time to fall asleep, and enhancing the depth of sleep.

SCIENTIFIC INSIGHTS

The chapter presented compelling scientific evidence showing that meditation activates the parasympathetic nervous system, promoting the 'rest and digest' state essential for restorative sleep.

Research findings were discussed to establish the effectiveness of meditation in improving sleep patterns and overall sleep quality.

PRACTICAL MEDITATION TECHNIQUES FOR SLEEP

We provided practical tips and detailed guides on various meditation routines specifically designed for better sleep.

Techniques like guided sleep meditation, body scan, and breath-focused meditation were explored, offering readers accessible methods to incorporate into their nightly routines.

ALEX'S TRANSFORMATION

Through Alex's journey, we witnessed the real-life impact of integrating meditation into sleep routines. His story of overcoming sleep disturbances and the subsequent improvements in his health, mood, and energy levels served as a relatable and inspiring example of the changes that are possible.

SUMMARY AND PREPARATION FOR CHAPTER 4

In Chapter 3, we embarked on an explorative journey to understand the profound connection between sleep, meditation, and aging. This chapter has illuminated key insights and practical strategies that underscore the transformative power of quality sleep and how meditation serves as a vital tool in achieving it. Let's recap the pivotal themes and prepare for the journey ahead in the next chapter.

As we close this chapter, our understanding of the interplay between sleep, meditation, and aging has deepened, offering new perspectives on how to nurture our well-being. But our exploration doesn't end here. In the next chapter, The Fountain of Youth, we will shift our focus to the emotional realm.

Emotions play a pivotal role in our overall health and aging process. The upcoming chapter will delve into how meditation influences our emotional well-being, helping to maintain a youthful spirit and a balanced life.

We will explore meditation's role in managing emotions, reducing stress, and enhancing resilience. Through practical advice, scientific insights, and real-life stories, we will discover how mastering our emotional landscape through meditation can lead to a more harmonious, fulfilling, and age-defying life.

Join us in the next chapter as we uncover the secrets to emotional wellness and longevity, further unlocking the full potential of meditation in our journey toward a healthier, more vibrant life.

Chapter 4
The Fountain Of Youth: Finding Emotional Balance

Introduction

Emotion is a complex psychological state that involves a range of feelings, such as happiness, sadness, anger, fear, and love, among others. Emotions are often accompanied by physiological changes, such as changes in heart rate, breathing, and muscle tension. They can be triggered by internal or external stimuli and can be expressed through a variety of behaviors, including facial expressions, body language, and tone of voice.

Emotions play an important role in our lives, influencing our thoughts, behaviors, and social interactions. They can be both positive and negative and can be experienced in varying intensities. Understanding and managing our emotions is an essential part of our overall well-being.

As we age, maintaining emotional balance becomes increasingly important, not only for mental well-being but also for physical health.

The Impact Of Meditation On Emotional Health

Meditation has long been celebrated for its ability to foster a deep sense of inner peace and emotional stability. It offers a unique pathway to understand and manage our emotions, leading to a more balanced and harmonious life.

REDUCING STRESS AND ANXIETY

Regular meditation practice has been shown to significantly lower levels of stress and anxiety. By focusing on the present moment and cultivating a non-judgmental attitude, meditation helps in breaking the cycle of chronic stress, which is often the root of emotional imbalance.

ENHANCING EMOTIONAL RESILIENCE

Meditation strengthens emotional resilience, empowering individuals to handle life's challenges with more composure and less reactivity.

This resilience is key to maintaining emotional balance, particularly in the face of the physical and psychological changes that accompany aging.

PROMOTING MINDFULNESS AND SELF-AWARENESS

Meditation enhances mindfulness, which in turn fosters greater self-awareness. This awareness is crucial for recognizing and regulating emotional responses, allowing for more thoughtful and measured reactions to situations.

MOOD AND REDUCING DEPRESSION

Regular meditation practice has been linked with increased levels of serotonin, often referred to as the 'happiness hormone.'

This increase can lead to improved mood and a significant reduction in symptoms of depression, which are common in the aging population.

CULTIVATING EMOTIONAL INTELLIGENCE

Meditation enhances the ability to understand and manage not only one's emotions but also those of others. This heightened emotional intelligence facilitates better interpersonal relationships and social interactions, which are crucial for mental well-being in later life.

STRESS-INDUCED AGING AND MEDITATION

Chronic stress accelerates the aging process by affecting cellular health, including telomere length and inflammation levels. Meditation, by mitigating stress, can help slow down these aging markers, contributing to both emotional and physical longevity.

EMOTION-FOCUSED MEDITATION PRACTICES AND TIPS

To cultivate emotional balance through meditation, consider incorporating the following practices into your routine:

MINDFULNESS MEDITATION

Practice observing your thoughts and emotions without judgment. Sit quietly and focus on your breath, allowing your emotions to surface and pass without getting attached to them.

FOCUSED BREATHING TECHNIQUES

Use breathing exercises to center your mind and calm your emotions. Techniques like deep belly breathing or alternate nostril breathing can be particularly effective.

GUIDED IMAGERY MEDITATION

This involves visualizing calming and peaceful images or scenarios to evoke positive emotions and relaxation. Guided imagery can be particularly effective in managing mood swings and emotional stress.

JOURNALING POST-MEDITATION

After meditation, spend a few minutes journaling your thoughts and feelings. This practice can provide deeper insights into your emotional state and help in processing complex emotions.

YOGA AND MEDITATION COMBINATION

Incorporating gentle yoga poses with meditation can enhance the emotional benefits. Yoga prepares the body and mind for meditation, making it easier to achieve a deeper state of relaxation.

GROUP MEDITATION SESSIONS

Participating in group meditation can create a sense of community and shared experience, which is beneficial for emotional health. These sessions can provide support and motivation, especially for those dealing with loneliness or isolation.

CASE STUDY 4:
EMOTIONAL REJUVENATION THROUGH MEDITATION

Maria, a 55-year-old teacher, found herself at a crossroads in life, grappling with the emotional upheavals that often accompany midlife transitions. As her children embarked on their own journeys, leaving the family home, and as she navigated the physical and emotional changes of menopause, Maria faced feelings of anxiety, loss, and a sense of uncertainty about the future.

BEGINNING OF MARIA'S MEDITATION JOURNEY

Maria's introduction to meditation came at a time when her emotional well-being was at its lowest. She sought a way to cope with her swirling emotions and found solace in the practice of mindfulness meditation. Initially, it was challenging for her to sit still and confront her feelings, but she persisted, learning to observe her emotions without judgment or overreaction.

SIGNIFICANT SHIFT IN EMOTIONAL STATE

Over weeks and months of consistent practice, Maria began to experience a significant shift in her emotional state. The constant anxiety that had been her companion started to dissipate. She found herself handling stressful situations with a newfound calmness and responding to changes in her life with a sense of serenity and acceptance rather than fear and resistance.

DEEPENING HER PRACTICE

As Maria's journey with meditation deepened, she explored various forms, including loving-kindness meditation, which had a profound effect on her interactions with others.

She noticed a growing sense of compassion and empathy, first towards herself and then extending outward to others. This practice helped her rebuild strained relationships and foster a stronger connection with those around her.

EXPANDED BENEFITS IN HER LIFE

- **IMPROVED RELATIONSHIPS:**
  Maria's increased emotional stability had a ripple effect on her relationships. With her family, she became more understanding and

patient. Her interactions with friends and colleagues grew richer and more fulfilling. She became known as someone who radiates warmth and understanding.

- **GREATER COPING SKILLS:**
Maria's enhanced resilience was evident in how she approached life's challenges. Where once small setbacks would have derailed her, she now approached them with a sense of clarity and calm. She developed a perspective that allowed her to see challenges as opportunities for growth rather than insurmountable obstacles.

- **PHYSICAL HEALTH IMPROVEMENTS:**
Perhaps most surprisingly, the changes in Maria's emotional state began to manifest physically. The chronic headaches that had plagued her, a physical manifestation of her stress, became less frequent. Her energy levels improved, and she found herself engaging in activities she had previously avoided due to fatigue.

REDISCOVERING JOY AND PURPOSE

Maria's meditation journey led her to rediscover joy and purpose in her life. She found pleasure in small moments – the quiet of early morning, the laughter of her students, the beauty of nature.

She began to pursue interests that she had long set aside, finding that with her newfound energy and perspective, she was eager to explore and experience new things.

SHARING HER EXPERIENCE

Inspired by her transformation, Maria started sharing her experiences with meditation. She began leading short meditation sessions at her school for fellow teachers, providing them with tools to manage their own stress and emotional challenges. Her story became one of inspiration within her community, showing others that it's never too late to seek change and find balance.

Maria's story is a testament to the power of meditation in transforming not just the mind but the entire being. Her journey from a state of emotional turmoil to one of balance and fulfillment illustrates the profound impact that regular meditation can have.

It serves as a reminder that emotional health is deeply interconnected with our overall well-being and that taking steps to nurture our emotional self is crucial, especially as we navigate the complex journey of aging.

CONCLUSION FOR CHAPTER 4: THE ELIXIR WITHIN

In the exploration of Chapter 4, we've delved into the heart of ageless living—a journey guided by the pursuit of emotional balance.

Through the practice of mindfulness and the transformative power of meditation, we've unearthed the truth that the essence of youth resides within us, waiting to be rediscovered.

Our emotional well-being is the linchpin to ageless living, and we've learned that it's not about erasing the passage of time but embracing it with grace and presence. The inner oasis of tranquillity is where we find the elixir of vitality, and it's in this space that the secrets of ageless living are unveiled.

As we conclude this chapter, let us remember that agelessness is not a destination but a state of being. With each mindful breath, we nurture the ageless spirit within, and in the chapters ahead, we'll continue to explore the pathways to a life that resonates with vitality, serenity, and the timeless essence of youth.

Chapter Key Points

MEDITATION AS A CATALYST FOR EMOTIONAL HEALTH

At the outset, we explored how meditation significantly reduces stress and anxiety, fostering an inner sense of peace and balance. This decrease in emotional turmoil not only enhances our emotional well-being but also has beneficial ripple effects on our physical health, particularly crucial as we navigate the aging process.

BUILDING EMOTIONAL RESILIENCE

A key focus of our discussion was on meditation's capacity to strengthen emotional resilience. This resilience allows individuals to face the inevitable challenges and fluctuations of life with greater poise and awareness, essential for maintaining emotional steadiness in the face of aging's various challenges.

PROMOTING MINDFULNESS AND AWARENESS

We delved into the role of meditation in enhancing mindfulness, leading to deeper self-awareness. This increased awareness is crucial in recognizing, understanding, and regulating emotional responses, fostering more thoughtful and balanced reactions to life's situations.

PRACTICAL MEDITATION TECHNIQUES FOR EMOTIONAL WELL-BEING

The chapter provided valuable guidance on incorporating emotion-focused meditation practices into daily life. Techniques such as mindfulness meditation, loving-kindness meditation, and focused breathing were highlighted, offering accessible ways to nurture emotional health.

THE STORY OF TRANSFORMATION

Central to this chapter was Maria's inspiring story, which illustrated the profound effects of regular meditation on emotional rejuvenation. Her journey from emotional upheaval to a state of harmony and contentment exemplified the powerful changes achievable through dedicated meditation practice.as illuminated key insights and practical strategies that underscore the transformative power of quality sleep and how meditation serves as a vital tool in achieving it.

SUMMARY AND PREPARATION FOR CHAPTER 5

As we conclude this chapter, enriched with knowledge and insights on emotional balance, we prepare to delve into another critical aspect of well-being: cognitive health and brain function. In the next chapter, we will explore the role of meditation in supporting and enhancing cognitive abilities.

Understanding the connection between meditation and brain health is essential in our holistic approach to aging. The upcoming chapter will reveal how meditation can enhance memory, boost cognitive function, and foster mental sharpness, crucial for maintaining cognitive health as we age. Join us as we continue our exploration, uncovering the ways in which meditation can be a key to preserving mental acuity and cognitive vitality throughout life's journey.

Chapter 5
Brain Health: Meditation's Role In Cognitive Longevity

Introduction

As we delve deeper into the journey of aging and mental acuity, the crucial role of brain health becomes increasingly evident. In this chapter, we delve into understanding how meditation, a practice with roots deeply embedded in ancient traditions, serves as a vital tool for cognitive function and longevity.

The brain, a complex and dynamic organ, undergoes various changes as we age. These changes can significantly impact memory, focus, and overall cognitive abilities.

Meditation emerges not just as a method for achieving mental tranquility but as a critical ally in maintaining and enhancing brain health.

The aging process can lead to alterations in brain structure and function, often resulting in a gradual decline in cognitive abilities. However, emerging research suggests that certain lifestyle choices and practices, including meditation, can influence the rate and nature of these changes. Meditation's role in cognitive health is multifaceted, offering benefits that extend far beyond relaxation and stress relief.

In exploring the profound connection between meditation and brain health, we consider various aspects such as neuroplasticity, stress management, attention, and focus. We also explore how regular meditation practice can actively contribute to maintaining cognitive sharpness and potentially counteracting the natural cognitive decline that accompanies aging.

Meditation's Influence On Brain Health

Neuroplasticity and Meditation

Neuroplasticity, the brain's remarkable ability to form new neural connections and adapt, is a key factor in cognitive longevity. Meditation has been found to significantly influence neuroplasticity, leading to changes in brain structure and function.

These changes, particularly in areas related to learning, memory, and emotional processing, can counteract the natural decline in cognitive functions that accompany aging.

Studies have shown that regular meditators exhibit increased gray matter density in these critical brain regions, indicative of enhanced neuroplasticity.

COMBATTING STRESS-RELATED COGNITIVE DECLINE

Chronic stress exerts a detrimental impact on the brain, accelerating cognitive decline and heightening the risk of neurodegenerative diseases.

Meditation's ability to reduce stress is crucial in protecting the brain from these adverse effects. By mitigating the release of stress hormones like cortisol, meditation aids in preserving cognitive functions and maintaining overall brain health.

Moreover, meditation helps in regulating the body's stress response, promoting a more balanced neurological reaction to stressful situations.

IMPROVING FOCUS AND ATTENTION

The ability to maintain attention and focus tends to diminish with age, impacting daily functioning and quality of life. Meditation practices, particularly those emphasizing focused attention, have demonstrated significant improvements in these cognitive abilities.

Engaging in regular meditation trains the brain to concentrate better, enhancing cognitive functions such as attention span, problem-solving skills, and working memory. This training is crucial for older adults, as it can lead to improved cognitive performance and a more active, engaged life.

PRACTICAL TIPS: CREATING COGNITIVE ENHANCEMENT

To unlock the full potential of meditation and harness its cognitive benefits, it is highly recommended to integrate advanced techniques into your daily practice. These techniques are designed to deepen your meditation experience and enhance its effects on the brain. By incorporating mindfulness, visualization, and loving-kindness meditation into your daily routine, you can improve your emotional regulation, reduce stress levels, and ultimately boost your overall well-being. So, if you are looking to take your meditation practice to the next level and reap its full range of benefits, consider integrating these advanced techniques into your daily routine.

MINDFULNESS AND COGNITIVE TRAINING

Mindfulness meditation is about more than stress reduction; it's a practice that enhances cognitive awareness. Regular mindfulness practice can lead to improved mental clarity and cognitive flexibility, which are vital for cognitive health. This form of meditation encourages a focus on the present moment, allowing practitioners to observe their thoughts and feelings without judgment, leading to a deeper understanding of their mental processes.

MANTRA MEDITATION FOR MEMORY

Mantra meditation involves focusing the mind on a particular word or phrase, which can aid in memory retention and recall. This practice helps concentrate the mind and can improve neural pathways associated with memory. The repetition of a mantra can serve as a mental exercise to strengthen cognitive functions, particularly in memory and recall.

YOGA-MEDITATION INTEGRATION

Combining yoga with meditation enhances the cognitive benefits of both practices. Yoga prepares the body and mind for deeper meditation, leading to improved mental focus and concentration.

The physical postures of yoga, coupled with breath control and meditation, create a holistic approach to cognitive enhancement.

GROUP MEDITATION FOR ENHANCED LEARNING

Participating in group meditation sessions offers additional cognitive benefits. The shared experience and collective learning in a group setting can stimulate new neural pathways and enhance brain plasticity. Group meditation can also provide a sense of community and support, which is beneficial for mental health and cognitive well-being.

LATEST SCIENTIFIC RESEARCH AND EXPERT OPINIONS

Recent studies in the field of neuroscience have illuminated the profound impact of meditation on the brain.

Notable neuroscientists, such as Dr. Sara Lazar of Harvard University, has shown through MRI scans that regular meditation can lead to increased gray matter in the hippocampus, known for its role in learning and memory, and in structures associated with self-awareness and introspection.

These findings are supported by other experts like Dr. Richard Davidson from the University of Wisconsin, who emphasize meditation's ability to reduce stress-related cortisol production, thereby protecting the brain from age-related decline.

This body of research presents a clear, evidence-based understanding of meditation's role in cognitive health and longevity, making it a compelling topic for both scientific and public interest.

DIVERSE MEDITATION PRACTICES FOR COGNITIVE HEALTH

This section explores various meditation styles and their unique benefits for cognitive health:

TRANSCENDENTAL MEDITATION (TM)

TM involves silently repeating a mantra for 20 minutes twice a day. It's known for reducing stress and anxiety, which are critical factors in cognitive health.

ZEN MEDITATION (ZAZEN)

This practice focuses on observing the breath and thoughts without attachment. Zazen can enhance concentration and mental discipline, key components for cognitive longevity.

VIPASSANA MEDITATION

Vipassana, or insight meditation, is about gaining a deep understanding of the true nature of reality. It enhances mindfulness and self-awareness, aiding cognitive and emotional processing.

INTERACTIVE ELEMENTS: GUIDED EXERCISES

Engage with interactive meditation exercises embedded in the text. These guided practices, tailored for cognitive enhancement, offer readers an experiential understanding of meditation's benefits.

Engaging with meditation exercises is a powerful way to gain a practical and experiential understanding of its cognitive benefits. This section provides readers with a series of interactive, guided meditation practices, focusing on mindfulness techniques that emphasize breath and body sensations. These practices are designed to enhance cognitive awareness, mental clarity, and provide a firsthand experience of meditation's impact on the brain.

GUIDED PRACTICE 1: MINDFUL BREATHING

FINDING A QUIET SPACE

Begin by finding a quiet and comfortable space where you will not be disturbed. Sit in a relaxed position, either on a chair with your feet flat on the ground or cross-legged on the floor. Keep your back straight but not rigid.

FOCUSING ON THE BREATH

Close your eyes and bring your attention to your breath. Notice the sensation of air entering and leaving your nostrils, or the rise and fall of your chest or abdomen as you breathe.

OBSERVING THE MIND

As you focus on your breath, you may notice that your mind begins to wander. This is normal. When you realize your attention has drifted, gently guide it back to your breath without judgment.

DURATION

Continue this practice for about 5-10 minutes to start. Over time, you can gradually increase the duration as you become more comfortable with the practice.

REFLECTING ON THE EXPERIENCE

After completing the exercise, take a moment to reflect on the experience. Observe any changes in your mental state, such as increased calmness or mental clarity.

GUIDED PRACTICE 2: BODY SCAN MEDITATION

PREPARATION

Lie down comfortably on your back with your arms at your sides, palms facing up. If lying down is uncomfortable, you can also do this practice sitting in a comfortable chair.

STARTING AT THE FEET

Bring your attention to your feet. Notice any sensations you feel - warmth, coolness, pressure, tingling, or perhaps nothing at all. Acknowledge these sensations without judgment.

PROGRESSING UPWARDS

Slowly move your attention up through your body - to your ankles, calves, knees, thighs, hips, abdomen, chest, back, shoulders, arms, hands, neck, and finally to your head. Spend a few moments at each part of your body, observing any sensations or feelings that arise.

MINDFUL OBSERVATION

If your mind wanders or if you notice discomfort or tension in a part of your body, acknowledge it without judgment and gently bring your attention back to the body scan.

COMPLETING THE PRACTICE

Once you reach the top of your head, take a few deep breaths and gently open your eyes. Reflect on the sensations experienced throughout the body and any feelings of relaxation or release of tension.

GUIDED PRACTICE 3: MINDFUL OBSERVATION

SELECTING AN OBJECT

Choose a small object, like a stone, leaf, or even a household item. Sit comfortably and hold the object in your hands.

ENGAGING THE SENSES

Examine the object closely. Notice its color, texture, weight, temperature, and any other physical qualities. See if you can engage all your senses – sight, touch, and even smell.

MINDFUL ATTENTION

As you observe the object, notice any thoughts or feelings that arise. Are you making judgments about it, or are your thoughts drifting to other topics?

Whenever you become aware of your mind wandering, gently bring your attention back to observing the object.

DURATION AND REFLECTION

Continue this exercise for about 5-10 minutes. Afterwards, reflect on the experience and any insights about your thought patterns or how easily your mind may wander.

These guided practices are just the beginning of a journey into mindfulness meditation. The real transformative power of these practices lies in their regular application.

To further enhance cognitive awareness and clarity, consider integrating mindfulness into your daily activities. This could involve mindfully eating a meal, paying full attention while listening to someone, or simply observing your thoughts and sensations during a walk.

By incorporating these practices into your life, you begin to cultivate a heightened sense of awareness and presence, which is instrumental in enhancing cognitive functions and overall mental well-being.

These exercises serve not just as a method for relaxation but as a tool for profound cognitive and emotional growth.

VISUAL AIDS:
UNDERSTANDING THE BRAIN ON MEDITATION

ILLUSTRATIVE BRAIN PHYSIOLOGICAL RESPONSE TO MEDITATION

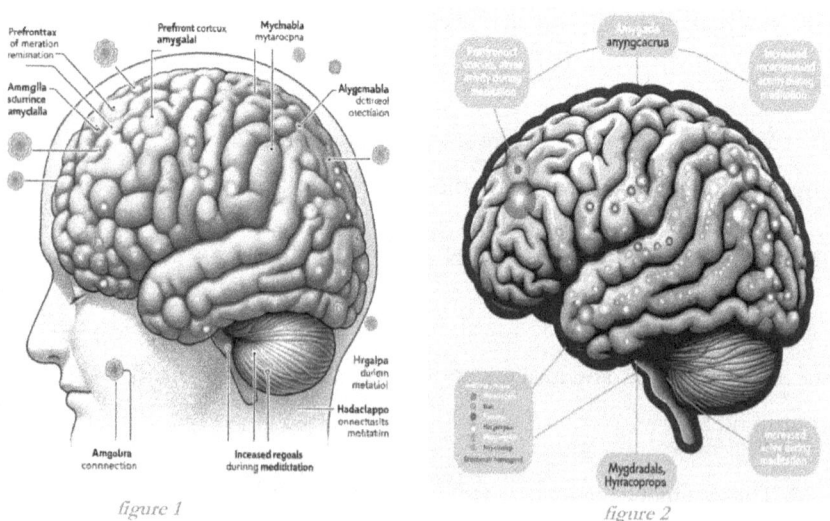

figure 1   *figure 2*

The provided illustrations offer a detailed view of the brain's active regions during meditation, using color-coding to denote areas of increased activity or connectivity. Key regions highlighted include the prefrontal cortex, amygdala, and hippocampus, each meticulously annotated for clear understanding.

The prefrontal cortex, known for its role in decision-making and self-regulation, shows heightened activity, which may explain the improved concentration and decision-making abilities observed in regular meditators.

Meanwhile, enhanced activity in the hippocampus, vital for memory and learning, suggests why meditation is linked to improved memory and cognitive function.

Understanding these changes is crucial, as it provides a neurological basis for the profound mental and emotional benefits attributed to regular meditation practice, highlighting its significance as a powerful tool for enhancing mental health and cognitive abilities.

ILLUSTRATIVE BENEFITS FOR THE BRAIN FROM MEDITATION

Meditation offers a myriad of benefits for the brain, succinctly captured in key points. It significantly reduces stress and anxiety by promoting relaxation. The practice enhances focus and concentration, making it easier to stay on task and maintain attention.

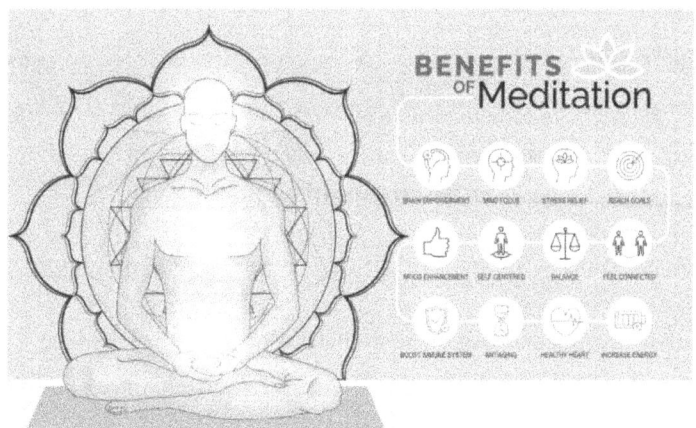

figure 3

Emotional regulation is another crucial benefit, as meditation aids in managing emotions more effectively. Mindfulness, heightened through regular practice, leads to an increased awareness of the present moment.

Additionally, meditation boosts memory and cognitive functions, aiding in information retention and processing. Over the long term, it promotes brain health and neuroplasticity, leading to a more adaptable and resilient mind.

ADDRESSING COMMON MISCONCEPTIONS

This section addresses and debunks prevalent myths about meditation and brain health, aiming to clarify the true scope and impact of meditation.

MISCONCEPTION 1: MEDITATION IS JUST RELAXATION

While meditation does induce relaxation, its benefits extend far beyond. Scientific research presented in this section shows how meditation enhances cognitive functions such as memory, attention, and problem-solving skills.

MISCONCEPTION 2: BENEFITS ARE ONLY PSYCHOLOGICAL

While meditation's psychological benefits are well-documented, its physiological effects are equally significant. Studies highlight changes in brain structure, improved neural plasticity, and alterations in neurotransmitter levels, proving meditation's comprehensive impact.

MISCONCEPTION 3: IMMEDIATE RESULTS ARE EXPECTED

Another common myth is that meditation yields immediate results. This section explains that, like any skill, meditation's cognitive benefits are more pronounced and lasting with regular and sustained practice.

By dispelling these myths, the chapter provides a more accurate and comprehensive understanding of meditation's role in cognitive health.

Discussion On Long-Term Practice Of Meditation

The practice of meditation, when sustained over long periods, has profound implications for brain health and cognitive functioning. This comprehensive exploration delves into the lasting changes in brain structure and function that consistent meditation practice can induce, drawing on a wealth of research and scientific studies.

SUSTAINED COGNITIVE BENEFITS

Long-term meditators often exhibit better-preserved brain matter and cognitive function, particularly in areas crucial for memory, attention, and emotional regulation. This is not just anecdotal evidence but is supported by rigorous scientific research.

PRESERVATION OF BRAIN MATTER

A groundbreaking study published in the journal "Frontiers in Psychology" found that individuals who meditated regularly showed less age-related decline in brain volume. Unlike the control group, long-term meditators maintained more gray matter volume, particularly in regions associated with cognitive processing and emotional regulation.

ENHANCED MEMORY AND ATTENTION

Regular meditation has been linked to improved performance in memory and attention tasks. Research published in "Consciousness and Cognition" demonstrated that participants who engaged in long-term meditation practices had better scores on tests of visual memory, sustained attention, and concentration.

EMOTIONAL REGULATION

The benefits of meditation extend to emotional health as well. Studies have shown that long-term meditation can lead to changes in brain regions related to emotional regulation, such as the amygdala, resulting in a more balanced and less reactive emotional response to stressors.

NEUROPLASTICITY OVER TIME

Neuroplasticity, the brain's ability to change and adapt throughout life, is significantly enhanced through prolonged meditation practice.

ENHANCING BRAIN PLASTICITY

A study from the "Journal of Neuroscience" reported that regular meditation contributes to increased neuroplasticity, leading to improved cognitive resilience and adaptability.

This is particularly evident in the prefrontal cortex, a region associated with higher-order thinking and decision-making.

CREATING NEW NEURAL PATHWAYS

Consistent meditation practice encourages the formation of new neural connections.

Research indicates that meditators often show increased connectivity between different brain regions, facilitating more efficient brain function and improved cognitive abilities.

REINFORCING LEARNING AND MEMORY

Meditation's impact on the hippocampus, the center for learning and memory in the brain, is notable.

Studies have found that meditators have more robust hippocampal structures, which correlates with enhanced memory and learning abilities.

AGING AND MEDITATION

Meditation's impact on the aging brain is an area of growing interest among neuroscientists.

MAINTAINING COGNITIVE FUNCTION

Research has indicated that meditation can play a significant role in maintaining cognitive function in older adults. A study in "NeuroImage" found that older individuals who engaged in regular meditation showed signs of slower cognitive decline compared to those who did not meditate.

DELAYING AGE-RELATED COGNITIVE DISORDERS

There is emerging evidence suggesting that meditation may delay the onset of age-related cognitive disorders such as Alzheimer's disease. This is thought to be due to meditation's ability to reduce stress, a known risk factor for Alzheimer's, and its role in enhancing brain plasticity.

ENHANCING MENTAL CLARITY IN OLDER ADULTS

Consistent meditation practice is associated with enhanced mental clarity and focus in older adults. This is supported by studies showing improved attention spans and problem-solving skills in older individuals who meditate regularly.

The evidence presented in this discussion underscores the powerful and lasting impact that consistent meditation practice can have on brain health. From preserving brain matter and enhancing cognitive functions to improving neuroplasticity and potentially delaying age-related cognitive decline, the benefits of sustained meditation are clear and significant.

These findings not only highlight the importance of meditation as a tool for cognitive maintenance and enhancement but also suggest its potential as a non-pharmacological intervention for aging-related cognitive decline. As research in this field continues to evolve, the understanding and appreciation of meditation's role in promoting long-term brain health are likely to deepen further.

Incorporating meditation into daily life, regardless of age, can be a proactive approach to maintaining cognitive vitality and overall brain health.

As we continue to unravel the complexities of the human brain and the impacts of our lifestyles upon it, meditation stands out as a simple yet profoundly effective practice for nurturing our cognitive well-being.

LIFESTYLE INTEGRATION: MAKING MEDITATION ACCESSIBLE

In the hustle and bustle of modern life, finding time and space for meditation can seem challenging. However, the beauty of meditation lies in its adaptability to different lifestyles and personal circumstances.

This section offers practical advice on integrating meditation into various life stages and situations, demonstrating how this age-old practice can be tailored to meet diverse needs.

FOR BUSY PROFESSIONALS

Professionals juggling demanding careers and personal commitments often find themselves grappling with high stress and limited time.

Here are some strategies to weave meditation into a busy schedule:

- **SHORT, FOCUSED MEDITATIONS**
  Time constraints shouldn't be a barrier to meditation. Short sessions, even five to ten minutes long, can be highly effective. Techniques like focused breathing or a quick body scan can be done almost anywhere – at your desk, during a commute, or between meetings.

- **MINDFULNESS IN DAILY TASKS**
  Turn everyday activities into meditative exercises. This could involve being fully present and mindful while drinking a cup of coffee, walking to work, or even during routine work tasks. By focusing completely on the task at hand, you cultivate mindfulness that can help in stress reduction and mental clarity.

- **UTILIZING APPS FOR GUIDED SESSIONS**
  Leverage technology to aid your practice. Meditation apps like Headspace, Calm, and Insight Timer offer guided sessions that can be squeezed into any part of the day. Many of these apps also provide specialized sessions for work-related stress, sleep, and focus.

- **SCHEDULED MEDITATION BREAKS**
  Just as you schedule meetings, pencil in meditation breaks. These scheduled pauses can provide a much-needed mental reset, improving productivity and creativity.

- **MINDFUL MEETINGS**
  Begin meetings with a minute or two of silent meditation. This practice can center the group, leading to more focused and productive discussions.

FOR RETIREES

Retirement brings a change in pace and lifestyle, offering an opportunity to delve deeper into meditation:

- **GROUP MEDITATION SESSIONS**
  Joining a meditation group can provide social interaction and a sense of community. Group sessions can be particularly motivating and enriching, providing shared experiences and learning.

- **LONGER MINDFULNESS PRACTICES**
  With more time at hand, retirees can engage in longer meditation sessions. This could involve more extended periods of sitting meditation, mindful walking, or engaging in mindfulness-based activities like gardening or painting.

- **MEDITATION FOR WELL-BEING IN RETIREMENT**
  Meditation can be particularly beneficial in addressing the emotional and psychological changes that come with retirement. Practices focusing on gratitude, acceptance, and compassion can enhance overall well-being.

- **TEACHING AND SHARING**
  Retirement can be an excellent time to share your meditation experience with others, perhaps by teaching family members or volunteering to lead sessions in community centers.

FOR INDIVIDUALS WITH HEALTH CONDITIONS

For those dealing with health conditions, meditation can be a valuable tool for managing stress and enhancing physical and mental health:

- **MEDITATION FOR STRESS MANAGEMENT**
  Chronic health conditions often bring added stress. Meditation can help manage this stress, which in turn can have a positive impact

on physical health. Practices like guided imagery or progressive muscle relaxation can be particularly beneficial

- **GENTLE YOGA-MEDITATION COMBINATIONS**
  Combining gentle yoga with meditation can be helpful for those with physical limitations. Yoga can aid in maintaining physical flexibility and strength, while meditation can help in coping with pain and illness.

- **BREATH AWARENESS PRACTICES**
  Focusing on the breath can be a simple yet effective way to meditate, especially for those who may find it challenging to engage in more physical forms of meditation. Breath awareness helps in cultivating a sense of calm and can be practiced in any comfortable position.

- **GUIDED MEDITATION FOR SPECIFIC CONDITIONS**
  Many meditation resources offer guided sessions targeted at specific health conditions, such as pain management, heart health, or insomnia.

- **MINDFULNESS IN TREATMENT AND RECOVERY:**
  Integrating mindfulness into treatment regimens and recovery processes can improve outcomes.

The versatility and adaptability of meditation make it an accessible practice for people from all walks of life. Whether you are a busy professional, a retiree, or someone managing a health condition, meditation can be tailored to fit your specific lifestyle and needs.

By integrating meditation into your daily routine, you open up a world of enhanced mental clarity, stress reduction, and overall well-being. As each person's journey with meditation is unique, the key is to explore and find practices that resonate with you and your lifestyle, creating a sustainable and enriching meditation routine.

Case Study 5: An Elder's Journey With Meditation For Mental Sharpness

James, a 70-year-old retired teacher, faced the inevitable challenges of aging, particularly in maintaining his cognitive sharpness. Once a voracious reader and avid problem-solver, he found that his once-sharp mind began to show signs of slowing down. He struggled with memory lapses, found it harder to concentrate, and often felt a step slower in conversations. It wasn't just about forgetting where he left his keys; it was a pervasive feeling that his mental edge was dulling.

DISCOVERING MEDITATION

James's introduction to meditation came during a community workshop. Initially skeptical, he was intrigued by the research presented on meditation's cognitive benefits.

With nothing to lose and much to potentially gain, he embarked on his meditation journey. He started with guided sessions, moving on to explore various forms, including mindfulness and focused attention practices.

EARLY STRUGGLES AND BREAKTHROUGHS

The early days of his practice were challenging. James grappled with a wandering mind, physical discomfort, and the nagging doubt of whether meditation was truly effective.

However, persistence led to breakthroughs. Gradually, he began to notice moments of clarity during his sessions, where his mind felt sharp and focused. These moments were fleeting at first but grew more prolonged and frequent over time.

INTEGRATING MEDITATION INTO DAILY LIFE

James made meditation a cornerstone of his daily routine. Mornings started with a session of mindfulness meditation, where he focused on his breath and observed his thoughts without judgment. Evenings were for focused attention practices, often involving concentration on a mantra or a visual object. This regular practice became something he looked forward to, a time of day when he felt most at peace and mentally alert.

COGNITIVE IMPROVEMENTS

A couple of months into his practice, James started noticing changes. His memory seemed more reliable; he could recall names and details he previously struggled with.

His concentration improved significantly, allowing him to read and engage in hobbies like chess with renewed vigor. Even more importantly, he found himself being more present in conversations, able to listen actively and respond with the sharp wit that was his hallmark.

REDISCOVERING OLD PASSIONS

Encouraged by his improving cognitive abilities, James began to rekindle old passions that required mental acuity. He joined a local chess club, a hobby he had abandoned years earlier, and found joy in the mental challenge it presented. He also started learning a new language, something he had always wanted to do but never felt mentally up to the task.

IMPACT ON MENTAL AND EMOTIONAL WELL-BEING

The benefits of James's meditation practice extended beyond cognitive enhancement. He experienced a profound sense of mental and emotional well-being.

The anxiety he often felt about aging and cognitive decline diminished. He felt more confident in his mental abilities and more optimistic about the future.

SHARING HIS EXPERIENCE

James became an advocate for meditation in his community, sharing his experience with peers. He led meditation groups at the local senior center, introducing others to the practice.

His story, relatable and inspiring, encouraged many to start their own journeys with meditation, transforming his role from a passive participant to an active proponent of mental wellness in later life.

REFLECTIONS ON THE JOURNEY

As James reflected on his meditation journey, he realized it was not just about cognitive preservation; it was about embracing a new chapter in life with mental vibrancy and clarity. Meditation had opened doors to a world where aging did not mean cognitive decline, but an opportunity for growth and learning.

James's story is a testament to the potential of meditation to profoundly impact cognitive health and overall quality of life. His journey from a state of concern about his cognitive decline to one of mental sharpness and vitality illustrates the transformative power of regular meditation practice.

It serves as a beacon of hope and a guide for others facing similar challenges, showing that it is never too late to begin, and the benefits can be life changing.

Conclusion For Chapter 5: Nurturing The Cognitive Fountain Of Youth

In Chapter 5, we embarked on a transformative voyage into the sphere of brain health, with meditation as our guiding light towards cognitive longevity.

Through the insights of mindfulness, we revealed the intricate interplay between a well-tended mind and its enduring brilliance.

Meditation's impact on cognitive longevity lies in its ability to cultivate a resilient, adaptable mind. It nurtures cognitive health by reducing stress, enhancing focus, and promoting neuroplasticity—the brain's capacity to form new neural connections.

These transformations empower us to harness the boundless potential of our intellect, offering a cognitive fountain of youth that transcends the passage of time.

As we conclude this chapter, let us carry with us the profound understanding that agelessness extends to the brilliance of the mind.

In the chapters ahead, we'll delve deeper into the dimensions of ageless living, uncovering the timeless principles that guide us towards a life marked by boundless cognitive vitality and enduring youth.

Chapter Key Points

SUSTAINED COGNITIVE BENEFITS

We explored how long-term meditation leads to the preservation of brain matter and improved cognitive function, particularly in areas critical for memory, attention, and emotional regulation.

NEUROPLASTICITY OVER TIME

The chapter highlighted meditation's remarkable ability to enhance neuroplasticity. This ongoing brain adaptability contributes to improved cognitive resilience and adaptability, crucial for mental agility and health.

AGING AND MEDITATION

A significant focus was on how meditation positively impacts the aging brain, helping to maintain cognitive function and potentially delay the onset of age-related cognitive disorders.

PRACTICAL INTEGRATION

The chapter provided practical advice for integrating meditation into various lifestyles, catering to busy professionals, retirees, and individuals with health conditions, thus emphasizing meditation's flexibility and accessibility for all.

SUMMARY **A**ND **P**REPARATION **F**OR **C**HAPTER 6

This chapter provides a thorough exploration of how meditation can be instrumental in supporting brain health and cognitive longevity, complete with practical advice and a detailed case study, preparing the reader for the exploration of meditation's role in physical wellness in the next chapter.

The journey of James has illustrated that cognitive longevity is achievable and that meditation can be a key component in maintaining mental sharpness. As we reach the conclusion of Chapter 5, we have delved deeply into the transformative impact of sustained meditation practice on cognitive health and brain function.

This chapter has illuminated the profound changes that regular meditation can bring about in our brains, underscoring its significance not just as a tool for momentary relaxation, but as a powerful agent for long-term cognitive enhancement and well-being.

As we turn the page to our next chapter, we embark on an exploration of a different but equally vital aspect of well-being: the relationship between meditation and physical health.

In this upcoming chapter, we will examine how meditation can reduce inflammation, enhance immune function, and contribute to overall physical health. We'll explore scientific studies and personal narratives that showcase how meditation can be a key component in managing and improving physical health conditions. From understanding meditation's role in pain management to its effects on heart health and sleep quality, Chapter 6 aims to provide a holistic view of how meditation can be a cornerstone in nurturing not just the mind, but the body as well.

Chapter 6
Body and Mind:
Physical Wellness and
The Body's Reflection Of The Mind

Introduction

In this chapter, we embark on an exploration of the significant impact of meditation on physical wellness. Meditation, often regarded primarily as a tool for mental and emotional well-being, also possesses far-reaching effects on the body. We'll examine how this ancient practice, rooted in mental discipline, translates into numerous physical health benefits, bridging the gap between mental practice and physical health.

The Science Of Meditation And Physical Health

Meditation's role in enhancing physical health is supported by a growing body of scientific research. The following are key areas where meditation has shown significant impact:

STRESS REDUCTION AND ITS PHYSICAL BENEFITS

Chronic stress is a major contributor to a host of physical health issues, including hypertension, heart disease, and weakened immune function.

Meditation's ability to reduce stress is not just mentally liberating but also physically beneficial. By lowering the body's stress responses, meditation helps mitigate these risks, leading to better overall health.

ENHANCING IMMUNE FUNCTION

The influence of meditation on the immune system is a remarkable area of study. Research, such as a study published in "Psychosomatic Medicine," has shown that mindfulness meditation can boost the immune response, exemplified by increased antibody production following vaccination. This suggests that meditation plays a role in bolstering the body's defense mechanisms.

IMPACT ON HEART HEALTH

Cardiovascular health is another area where meditation has shown significant benefits. Studies, including those published in the "Journal of the American Heart Association," indicate that regular meditation can lower blood pressure, a key risk factor in heart disease.

This reduction in blood pressure and improvement in heart rate variability points to meditation's protective role in heart health.

AIDING PAIN MANAGEMENT

Meditation's efficacy in managing chronic pain represents a major breakthrough in pain management. Research in "JAMA Internal Medicine" revealed that mindfulness meditation can lead to significant reductions in pain symptoms and enhancements in the quality of life for individuals suffering from chronic pain conditions.

ANTI-AGING PROPERTIES

At the cellular level, meditation may contribute to slowing down the aging process. Studies have indicated that meditation can preserve the length of telomeres, the protective caps at the ends of chromosomes. Telomeres serve as indicators of biological aging, and their preservation through meditation suggests a potential for slowing the aging process at a cellular level.

IMPROVING GASTROINTESTINAL HEALTH

Meditation has been shown to improve symptoms associated with gastrointestinal disorders. By reducing stress, which is a known exacerbating factor for conditions like irritable bowel syndrome (IBS) and inflammatory bowel disease (IBD), meditation can lead to improved gut health and digestion.

ENHANCING RESPIRATORY FUNCTION

For those with respiratory conditions such as asthma or COPD, meditation can improve respiratory function. Techniques like deep breathing in meditation help increase lung capacity and improve overall respiratory efficiency.

MEDITATION AND SLEEP

Meditation's role in enhancing sleep quality directly impacts physical health. Quality sleep is essential for physical repair, hormonal balance, and overall health. By improving sleep patterns, meditation contributes to better physical health.

REDUCING INFLAMMATION

Chronic inflammation is linked to many diseases, including arthritis, diabetes, and cancer. Meditation's stress-reducing properties can lower inflammation in the body, thus reducing the risk of these conditions.

IMPACT ON HORMONAL BALANCE

Meditation can influence hormonal balance in the body, leading to beneficial effects on conditions influenced by hormonal changes, such as menopause or thyroid disorders.

PRACTICAL TIPS: MEDITATIONS FOR PHYSICAL WELLNESS

In the pursuit of physical wellness, meditation emerges as a powerful tool with multifaceted benefits. While some techniques may overlap with those aimed at mental and emotional well-being, specific practices can be particularly effective for enhancing physical health.

This section offers comprehensive and intriguing tips, presented in an engaging style, to guide you in integrating meditation into your journey towards physical wellness.

1. BODY SCAN MEDITATION FOR PHYSICAL AWARENESS AND RELAXATION

Body scan meditation is a technique that promotes heightened awareness and relaxation of the physical body. It involves mentally scanning your body from head to toe, observing sensations without judgment.

- **HOW TO PRACTICE**

    Lie down or sit in a comfortable position. Close your eyes and start focusing on your breath. Then, gradually shift your attention to the top of your head and slowly move down to your toes, noticing any tension, pain, or discomfort.

- **BENEFITS**

  This practice can help in identifying areas of physical tension and promoting relaxation, essential for overall physical health. It's particularly beneficial for those who hold stress in their muscles and can aid in pain management.

2. BREATH-FOCUSED MEDITATION FOR RESPIRATORY HEALTH

Breathing exercises are central to many meditation practices, and they can significantly improve respiratory function and oxygenation of the body.

- **HOW TO PRACTICE**

  Sit or lie in a comfortable position. Focus on your breathing, observing the natural inhalation and exhalation. You can also practice deep breathing, where you inhale slowly through your nose, hold your breath for a few seconds, and exhale slowly through your mouth.

- **BENEFITS**

  This practice enhances lung capacity and efficiency, which is beneficial for overall vitality and can be particularly helpful for those with respiratory conditions.

3. WALKING MEDITATION FOR MIND-BODY COORDINATION

Walking meditation combines physical activity with mindful awareness, offering a unique way to integrate meditation into movement.

- **HOW TO PRACTICE**

  Choose a quiet and safe place to walk. Focus on the experience of walking, paying attention to the sensation of your feet touching the ground and the rhythm of your steps.

- **BENEFITS**

  This form of meditation is excellent for those who find stillness challenging. It improves mind-body coordination, balances energy levels, and provides gentle physical exercise.

4. TAI CHI AND QIGONG: MOVING MEDITATION FOR PHYSICAL WELLNESS

Tai Chi and Qigong are ancient practices that combine meditation, movement, and breathing. They can be considered a form of moving meditation.

- **HOW TO PRACTICE**

  These practices involve slow, graceful movements synchronized with breath control. You can join a class or follow online tutorials to learn the basics.

- **BENEFITS**

  Tai Chi and Qigong enhance physical balance, flexibility, and strength. They also improve circulation and can be particularly beneficial for older adults for fall prevention and general vitality.

5. GUIDED IMAGERY MEDITATION FOR PAIN MANAGEMENT

Guided imagery is a powerful meditation technique for managing pain and enhancing the body's healing process.

- **HOW TO PRACTICE**

    Find a comfortable place to relax. Listen to a guided imagery recording or visualize a peaceful and healing environment. Imagine your pain or discomfort being washed away by healing energy or light.

- **BENEFITS**

    This technique can alter the perception of pain and is useful in chronic pain management. It also promotes a sense of wellbeing and relaxation.

6. YOGA NIDRA FOR DEEP RELAXATION AND HEALING

Yoga Nidra, also known as yogic sleep, is a deep relaxation technique with roots in yoga.

- **HOW TO PRACTICE**

    Lie down comfortably. Follow a guided Yoga Nidra session, which will lead you through a systematic relaxation of the entire body, often accompanied by visualization and intention setting.

- **BENEFITS**

    Yoga Nidra is known for its capacity to induce deep relaxation, reduce stress, and aid in sleep disorders. It also supports the body's healing processes and can be beneficial in recovery from illness or injury.

7. CHAKRA MEDITATION FOR ENERGY BALANCE

Chakra meditation focuses on the body's energy centers and can be a useful practice for balancing and enhancing physical energy.

- **HOW TO PRACTICE**

  Sit comfortably and focus on each of the body's seven chakras, from the base of the spine to the crown of the head, visualizing energy flowing smoothly through each center.

- **BENEFITS**

  This practice can help in releasing energy blockages, which can contribute to various physical ailments. It promotes a sense of energetic balance and harmony in the body.

8. LAUGHTER MEDITATION FOR PHYSICAL AND MENTAL HEALTH

Laughter meditation combines unconditional laughter with deep breathing exercises, offering a unique approach to wellness.

- **HOW TO PRACTICE**

  Start with gentle breathing exercises, then allow yourself to laugh without relying on humor or jokes. Let the laughter flow naturally, even if it starts as forced.

- **BENEFITS**

  Laughter boosts the immune system, releases endorphins, reduces stress hormones, and provides a fun and effective way to improve overall health.

9. PROGRESSIVE MUSCLE RELAXATION FOR TENSION RELEASE

Progressive muscle relaxation involves tensing and relaxing different muscle groups, promoting physical relaxation and stress relief.

- **HOW TO PRACTICE**

  Lie down or sit in a comfortable chair. Tense each muscle group for a few seconds and then relax it, starting from the toes and moving up to the head.

- **BENEFITS**

    This technique is effective in reducing physical tension, which can lead to various health issues. It's especially beneficial for those who experience stress-related muscle tension.

CASE STUDY 6: A HEALTH TRANSFORMATION STORY

THE BEGINNING

Mark, a 58-year-old accountant, found himself at a crossroads in terms of his health. Overweight, with high blood pressure and chronic back pain, he was the epitome of a stressful and sedentary lifestyle. Mark's diet was poor, consisting mainly of fast food and processed snacks.

He had little to no physical activity, and his sleep patterns were irregular, often disrupted by his back pain and stress-related insomnia.

THE WAKE-UP CALL

The turning point came during a routine health checkup when his doctor expressed serious concerns about his cardiovascular health and the risk of diabetes. This was a wake-up call for Mark. He realized that if he didn't change his lifestyle, he might not be around to see his grandchildren grow up.

DISCOVERING MEDITATION

Mark's journey into meditation began somewhat by chance. A friend invited him to a local meditation class, suggesting it might help with his stress and sleep issues.

Skeptical but desperate for change, Mark attended his first session. It was challenging at first; he struggled to sit still, his mind was constantly wandering, and he felt out of place.

But there was something about the quiet, the focus on breathing, and the gentle guidance of the instructor that resonated with him. He decided to give it a more serious try and started attending classes regularly.

THE FIRST STEPS OF CHANGE

As Mark incorporated meditation into his daily routine, he noticed subtle changes. His sleep started to improve; he fell asleep more quickly and woke up feeling more rested. His stress levels began to drop, and he found himself reacting more calmly in situations that would have previously sent his blood pressure soaring.

Encouraged by these changes, Mark started making other lifestyle adjustments. He began to pay more attention to his diet, opting for healthier choices and reducing his intake of processed foods. He also started walking every day, gradually increasing his distance and pace.

DEEPENING THE PRACTICE

As his meditation practice deepened, so did Mark's understanding of his body and mind. He became more in tune with his physical sensations and emotional responses. Meditation sessions became a time for him to connect with himself, to reflect, and to find a sense of peace.

Mark explored different forms of meditation, including mindfulness, loving-kindness, and body scan meditations. Each type offered unique benefits – mindfulness helped him stay present, loving-kindness opened his heart to self-compassion, and body scans brought awareness to areas of his body that needed care.

PHYSICAL HEALTH IMPROVEMENTS

After six months, the physical changes in Mark were evident. He had lost a significant amount of weight, his blood pressure had normalized, and his back pain had reduced considerably. His doctor was amazed at the transformation and reduced his medication dosages.

Mark felt like a new person. He was more energetic, his mood had improved, and he started enjoying activities he had avoided for years, like hiking and cycling. The back pain that had plagued him for so long was no longer a constant in his life.

THE RIPPLE EFFECT

Mark's health transformation had a ripple effect on his relationships. His family noticed the changes – not just in his appearance but in his demeanor. He was more engaged, happier, and more present.

Friends and colleagues began asking him about his secret, and he proudly shared his journey into meditation and lifestyle change.

SHARING HIS JOURNEY

Inspired by his own transformation, Mark started a meditation group at his workplace. He wanted to share the practice that had so profoundly impacted his life. The group met weekly, providing a space for employees to destress and learn meditation techniques.

REFLECTIONS AND LOOKING FORWARD

Looking back on his journey, Mark saw his initial health crisis as a blessing in disguise. It propelled him onto a path of self-discovery and holistic well-being. Meditation had been the catalyst for this change, teaching him the importance of taking care of both his mind and body.

Mark's story is a testament to the power of meditation in transforming not just mental health but physical health as well. His experience illustrates how incorporating meditation into daily life can lead to profound and lasting changes, fostering a healthier, more fulfilling lifestyle.

Conclusion For Chapter 6: The Power Of Mind-Body Unity

In the heart of Chapter 6, we've unearthed a profound truth: ageless living is an intricate tapestry woven from the threads of our physical well-being and the intimate dance it shares with our minds. This chapter has illuminated the undeniable connection between the vitality of our bodies and the tranquillity of our minds.

Here, we've learned that agelessness is not a solitary pursuit of superficial aesthetics but a profound journey of nurturing the synergy between our bodies and minds. Our bodies serve as canvases, mirroring the masterpieces painted by our mental and emotional states.

Through these revelations, we've gained the knowledge that agelessness is a profound symphony, where the harmonious union of physical and mental wellness takes center stage. It's the understanding that our bodies are not passive spectators but active participants in the grand performance of our lives.

As we move forward, let's carry with us the certainty that Chapter 6 has bestowed—a life marked by ageless vitality emerges when we acknowledge the inseparable connection between body and mind.

CHAPTER KEY POINTS

HOLISTIC IMPACT OF MEDITATION ON PHYSICAL HEALTH

We delved into how meditation transcends mental boundaries to positively affect physical well-being. The chapter emphasized meditation's role in reducing stress and its direct physical benefits, such as lowering blood pressure and improving heart health.

MEDITATION ENHANCING IMMUNE FUNCTION

We explored compelling research showing that meditation can boost the immune system, fortifying the body's natural defense mechanisms.

THE ROLE OF MEDITATION IN HEART HEALTH

The chapter highlighted studies suggesting that regular meditation practice can contribute significantly to cardiovascular health by reducing risk factors like hypertension.

MEDITATION AS AN EFFECTIVE TOOL FOR PAIN MANAGEMENT

We discussed how meditation can be a powerful ally in managing chronic pain, providing relief and improving the quality of life for those suffering from persistent pain conditions.

ANTI-AGING EFFECTS OF MEDITATION

The chapter presented fascinating insights into how meditation might slow the aging process at a cellular level, preserving telomere length and enhancing overall vitality.

MARK'S HEALTH TRANSFORMATION

Mark's inspiring story served as a practical example of how integrating meditation into daily life can lead to significant improvements in physical health, reinforcing the themes discussed throughout the chapter.

SUMMARY AND PREPARATION FOR CHAPTER 7

As we reach the end of our exploration into the profound effects of meditation on physical health, we take a moment to reflect on the significant insights gained. Our journey has illuminated how a practice often associated with mental and emotional well-being can extend its benefits into the physical realm. This exploration has highlighted the tangible physical advantages that meditation offers, transcending its traditional perception. Let's summarize the key themes we've discovered and anticipate the further exploration that awaits us.

Building on our understanding of the physical benefits of meditation, the next chapter will take us into the realm of emotional well-being.

Here, we will explore how meditation not only aids in managing stress and anxiety but also fosters deeper emotional intelligence, resilience, and overall happiness.

We will delve into practical meditation techniques and strategies that specifically target emotional health, backed by scientific research and anecdotal evidence. The upcoming chapter aims to provide a comprehensive guide on how meditation can be a transformative tool in achieving emotional harmony and stability, contributing to a more balanced and fulfilling life.

Chapter 7
Daily Integration: Weaving Meditation Into Daily Life For Ageless Living

Introduction

Meditation is a powerful tool that can help us lead a more fulfilling life, no matter what our age. It is not just a practice but a way of life that can bring about positive changes in our mental, emotional, and physical well-being. By integrating meditation into our daily routines, we can experience a sense of calm, balance, and inner peace that enhances our overall well-being and helps us lead a life of ageless living.

In this chapter, we delve into the art of seamlessly integrating meditation into everyday life. As we have explored throughout this journey, meditation is not just a practice but a way of living, offering countless benefits for mental, emotional, and physical health. This chapter focuses on how to embed meditation into the fabric of our daily routines, transforming it from a solitary practice into a holistic lifestyle for ageless living.

Understanding the Essence of Daily Integration

MEDITATION AS A LIFESTYLE

The first step in integrating meditation into daily life is to shift our perception of it from an isolated activity to a continuous, living practice. It's about cultivating mindfulness and presence in every action, from the moment we wake up to when we retire for the night.

CREATING A PERSONALIZED MEDITATION ROUTINE

Each individual's life rhythm is unique, and so should be their meditation practice. This section explores how to tailor a meditation routine that aligns with personal schedules, responsibilities, and preferences, ensuring it's both enjoyable and sustainable.

THE RIPPLE EFFECT OF MEDITATION

Integrating meditation into daily life has a compounding effect. We'll explore how small, consistent practices can lead to significant changes over time, impacting every aspect of our lives.

Practical Ways To Incorporate Meditation

MORNING RITUALS:

Begin the day with a meditation session, setting a calm and centered tone for the day ahead. This can be as simple as a few minutes of deep breathing or a full session of mindfulness practice.

MINDFUL COMMUTING

Transform commuting time into an opportunity for meditation. If using public transport, try mindfulness or loving-kindness meditation. If driving, focus on being fully present and aware of the surroundings, turning the journey into a meditative experience.

MEDITATION BREAKS AT WORK

Incorporate short meditation sessions during work breaks. This can be a 5-minute breathing exercise at your desk or a brief walk outside, practicing walking meditation.

MINDFUL EATING

Turn meals into a meditative experience by eating mindfully. Pay attention to the flavors, textures, and sensations of your food, eating slowly and appreciatively.

EVENING UNWIND

End the day with a meditation session to unwind and reflect. This could involve a body scan to relax, a gratitude meditation, or journaling post-meditation to consolidate insights.

INTEGRATING MEDITATION INTO PHYSICAL ACTIVITIES

YOGA AND MEDITATION SYNERGY

Combine yoga with meditation for a holistic mind-body practice. Engage in yoga as a form of moving meditation, focusing on breath and movement alignment.

MEDITATIVE WALKS IN NATURE

Regular walks in nature can be transformed into meditative experiences. Practice being present, observing the natural surroundings with full attention and appreciation.

GENTLE EXERCISE AND MEDITATION

Incorporate meditation into routine physical exercises, such as stretching or light aerobic exercises, enhancing the mind-body connection.

MEDITATION IN RELATIONSHIPS AND SOCIAL INTERACTIONS

LISTENING WITH PRESENCE

Practice mindful listening in your interactions. Give your full attention to the person speaking, fostering deeper connections, and understanding.

COMPASSION AND LOVING-KINDNESS PRACTICES

Regularly engage in loving-kindness meditation to cultivate compassion and empathy in your relationships.

GROUP MEDITATION

Participate in or organize group meditation sessions, fostering a sense of community and shared experience.

OVERCOMING CHALLENGES IN INTEGRATION

DEALING WITH RESISTANCE

Address common challenges like time constraints and distractions, offering solutions to overcome them.

STAYING MOTIVATED

Explore ways to maintain motivation and commitment to your meditation practice, including keeping a meditation journal, setting goals, and celebrating milestones.

LONG-TERM BENEFITS OF INTEGRATED MEDITATION PRACTICE

CULTIVATING A PEACEFUL MIND

Consistent meditation leads to a more peaceful and centered mind, reducing stress and enhancing overall well-being.

PHYSICAL HEALTH BENEFITS

Over time, the integration of meditation contributes to improved physical health, from better sleep to enhanced immune function and longevity.

EMOTIONAL AND MENTAL CLARITY

Regular meditation fosters emotional balance and mental clarity, aiding in decision-making and creative thinking.

SPIRITUAL GROWTH

Meditation opens the doors to deeper spiritual exploration and understanding, enriching one's sense of purpose and connection.

PRACTICAL TIPS: BUILDING A SUSTAINABLE MEDITATION PRACTICE

INTRODUCTION TO SUSTAINABLE MEDITATION PRACTICES

In the realm of meditation, sustainability is key. A consistent and enduring practice can lead to profound transformations in both mental and physical well-being.

This section focuses on practical and fresh tips to build a meditation practice that not only fits into your daily life but also evolves with you over time. We aim to offer insights that differ from what we've explored in previous chapters, providing new perspectives on cultivating a meditation habit that endures and adapts to life's changing rhythms.

UNDERSTANDING YOUR PERSONAL MEDITATION STYLE

IDENTIFYING YOUR MEDITATION PREFERENCES

Recognize that meditation is not one-size-fits-all. Begin by exploring various meditation styles – from silent mindfulness to guided visualizations, mantra-based practices, or movement meditations like Tai Chi or Qigong. Discover what resonates with you the most.

CUSTOMIZING YOUR PRACTICE

Adapt meditation practices to suit your personality, lifestyle, and current needs. If you're a morning person, consider a vibrant, energizing meditation practice to start your day. For night owls, a calming, reflective meditation in the evening might be more effective.

ESTABLISHING A ROUTINE

SETTING REALISTIC GOALS

Start with attainable goals. If sitting for 30 minutes daily seems overwhelming, begin with 5 or 10 minutes and gradually increase the duration.

CREATING A DEDICATED SPACE

Designate a specific area in your home as your meditation space. This doesn't have to be elaborate – a comfortable chair or cushion in a quiet corner is sufficient. The key is to have a space that mentally prepares you for your practice.

INTEGRATING MEDITATION INTO DAILY ACTIVITIES

Incorporate mindfulness into everyday tasks like showering, eating, or walking. Use these activities as opportunities to practice mindfulness, focusing on sensations and experiences.

USING TECHNOLOGY MINDFULLY

MEDITATION APPS AND ONLINE RESOURCES

Utilize technology to support your practice. Meditation apps can provide guided sessions, timers, and reminders. However, be mindful not to become overly reliant on these tools; use them as a supplement to your practice.

DIGITAL DETOXES

Regularly schedule digital detoxes to disconnect from electronic devices and clear your mind, creating space for deeper meditation.

OVERCOMING OBSTACLES

DEALING WITH DISTRACTIONS

Distractions are a natural part of life. When distracted during meditation, gently acknowledge the distraction and return your focus to your breath or chosen point of concentration.

EMBRACING IMPERFECTION

Some days, meditation might feel challenging or unproductive. Embrace these experiences as part of the journey. Meditation is not about achieving perfection but about continual growth and self-discovery.

CULTIVATING MINDFULNESS THROUGHOUT THE DAY

MINDFUL REMINDERS

Set reminders throughout the day to pause and check in with yourself. Use these moments to take a few deep breaths and center yourself.

MINDFUL EATING

Transform mealtimes into mindful experiences. Eat slowly and savor each bite, paying attention to flavors, textures, and your body's signals.

MINDFUL MOVEMENT

Engage in regular physical activity mindfully. Whether it's yoga, walking, or stretching, focus on your body's movements and sensations.

BUILDING A SUPPORTIVE COMMUNITY

JOINING MEDITATION GROUPS

Consider joining a meditation group or community. Practicing with others can provide motivation, support, and a sense of connection.

SHARING YOUR PRACTICE

Share your meditation experiences with friends or family. Discussing your journey can offer new insights and strengthen your commitment to the practice.

CONTINUING EDUCATION IN MEDITATION

WORKSHOPS AND RETREATS

Attend meditation workshops or retreats to deepen your practice. These can provide immersive experiences and opportunities to learn from experienced practitioners.

READING AND RESEARCH

Regularly read books, articles, and scientific studies on meditation to expand your understanding and keep your practice fresh.

MAKING MEDITATION A LIFELONG PRACTICE

REFLECTING ON YOUR JOURNEY

Periodically reflect on your meditation journey. Acknowledge your growth and the benefits you've experienced.

ADAPTING YOUR PRACTICE AS YOU CHANGE

As you evolve, so should your meditation practice. Be open to trying new techniques and adapting your practice to align with your current life stage and needs.

Case Study 7: Integrating Meditation Into A Lifestyle Introduction

Sarah, a 45-year-old marketing executive, found herself at a crossroads in life. Juggling a high-pressure job, family responsibilities, and an array of social commitments, she often felt overwhelmed, stressed, and disconnected from her true self. Her journey of integrating meditation into her lifestyle is a tale of transformation, resilience, and discovery.

THE CATALYST FOR CHANGE

Sarah's introduction to meditation came at a time when she felt her life was spiraling out of control. Chronic stress, irregular sleep patterns, and a lack of personal time were taking their toll. A chance encounter with a meditation workshop flier in a local café sparked her curiosity.

INITIAL SKEPTICISM AND FIRST STEPS

Initially skeptical, Sarah attended her first meditation class with a mixture of curiosity and apprehension. Her first few attempts at meditation were challenging. Her mind raced with thoughts, and she found it difficult to sit still. Despite these challenges, there was a glimmer of peace in those few moments of stillness that kept her coming back.

BUILDING A ROUTINE

Determined to give meditation a fair chance, Sarah started with short, daily sessions. She began with guided meditations, using apps and online resources to stay on track. Gradually, as she became more comfortable, she extended her meditation time and started exploring different types of practices, including mindfulness, loving-kindness, and body scan meditation.

OVERCOMING CHALLENGES

One of Sarah's biggest challenges was finding time for meditation. With a packed schedule, it often felt like there was no space for a meditation routine. She started waking up 30 minutes earlier to meditate, a decision that transformed her mornings from hectic to serene.

Another challenge was dealing with distractions. With a busy household, finding a quiet space was difficult. Sarah converted a small corner of her bedroom into her meditation space, signaling to her family that this was her time for peace and quiet.

EXPERIENCING THE BENEFITS

After several weeks, the benefits of meditation began to materialize in Sarah's life. Her sleep improved, and she felt more energized throughout the day. She noticed a decrease in her stress levels and found herself handling work pressures with more composure.

INTEGRATING MINDFULNESS INTO DAILY LIFE

Sarah started to weave mindfulness into her everyday activities. She practiced mindful eating, savoring her food rather than rushing through meals. Her daily walks became exercises in mindfulness, observing her surroundings and sensations with heightened awareness.

THE TRANSFORMATION

Months into her practice, Sarah's transformation was evident. Colleagues noticed her newfound calmness, her family appreciated her increased presence and patience, and she felt a deep sense of fulfillment. Meditation had become an integral part of her life, not just a practice but a way of living.

EXPANDING HER PRACTICE

Encouraged by her progress, Sarah began attending weekend meditation retreats, deepening her practice, and understanding. She explored different meditation traditions, expanding her knowledge.

SHARING THE JOURNEY

Inspired by her transformation, Sarah started a meditation group at work. She shared her journey with colleagues, encouraging them to explore meditation. This group became a space for collective growth, support, and learning.

REFLECTING ON THE JOURNEY

As Sarah reflected on her meditation journey, she realized how it had transformed not just her stress levels but her entire approach to life. She had become more mindful, more in tune with her needs, and more connected to the people around her.

FACING NEW CHALLENGES

Life continued to present challenges, but now Sarah had the tools to face them. When her company faced a crisis, she used meditation to maintain her clarity and focus. When personal issues arose, she found solace and strength in her practice.

EMBRACING LIFELONG LEARNING

Sarah viewed her meditation journey as a path of lifelong learning. She continued to explore new techniques, attend workshops, and read extensively on meditation and mindfulness.

Sarah's story is a powerful testament to the transformative power of integrating meditation into daily life. Her journey from a stressed executive to a mindful, centered individual underscores the profound impact that consistent meditation practice can have on one's lifestyle and well-being.

CHAPTER KEY POINTS:

PERSONALIZING YOUR MEDITATION PRACTICE

We emphasized the importance of identifying a meditation style that resonates with you and adapting it to fit your unique lifestyle, ensuring it remains enjoyable and sustainable.

ESTABLISHING A CONSISTENT ROUTINE

Setting realistic goals and creating a dedicated meditation space can help in establishing a consistent practice. Regular meditation sessions, whether in the morning or evening, can set a tone of calmness and balance for the day.

INTEGRATING MINDFULNESS INTO EVERYDAY ACTIVITIES

We explored how mindfulness can be woven into daily tasks, transforming mundane activities into moments of awareness and presence.

LEVERAGING TECHNOLOGY MINDFULLY

Utilizing digital tools like apps and online resources can support and enhance your practice, while also recognizing the importance of periodic digital detoxes.

BUILDING A SUPPORTIVE COMMUNITY

Engaging with meditation groups and sharing experiences with others can reinforce your practice and foster a sense of community.

ADAPTING TO LIFE'S CHANGES

We discussed the importance of evolving your meditation practice to align with life's changing circumstances, ensuring that it remains relevant and supportive.

Conclusion To Chapter 7: The Daily Art Of Agelessness

As we reach the culmination of Chapter 7, we're confronted with a profound truth—the art of ageless living isn't a distant aspiration, but a daily practice that transforms our lives.

This chapter has unveiled the significance of seamlessly integrating meditation into our daily routines. It's not merely a theoretical concept; it's a tangible gateway to enduring vitality and timeless youth.

In the essence of this chapter lies a crucial revelation: agelessness is not a remote ideal, but a present reality. It's the understanding that by infusing each moment with mindfulness, we create a life marked by wellness, serenity, and unwavering youth.

Summary And Preparation For Chapter 8

As we bring this chapter to a close, we take a moment to reflect on the essential insights and practices we've explored for integrating meditation into daily life. This chapter has been a comprehensive guide to making meditation an integral part of your lifestyle, a journey towards achieving ageless living through mindfulness and self-awareness.

In the next chapter, we will gracefully transition from the inner tranquility cultivated through meditation to the art of mindful eating, an essential component of nurturing both body and mind. Chapter 8 expands upon the foundation of mindfulness and self-awareness laid in Chapter 7, providing a comprehensive exploration of how the principles of mindfulness can be applied to our eating habits.

Just as we have learned to personalize meditation practices and integrate mindfulness into everyday activities, Chapter 8 will guide you through the journey of transforming your relationship with food. This chapter is not just about what we eat but how we eat, offering insights into how the act of eating can become a meditative and enriching

Chapter 8
The Art Of Mindful Eating: Nourishing Body And Mind

Introduction

Are you ready for the next step in our journey towards a youthful and ageless life? Welcome to the world of mindful eating, a practice that combines the principles of meditation with the way we nourish ourselves, and brings harmony to our mind, body, and soul. Get ready to embark on a journey that will revolutionize the way you eat, and ultimately, the way you live.

Picture this: a serene dining setting, where every morsel of food becomes a gateway to mindfulness. In today's world of fast-paced living and on-the-go meals, the concept of savoring each bite might seem like a distant dream. Yet, as we'll discover, mindful eating holds the potential to transform your relationship with food, elevate your overall well-being, and contribute to the radiant health and vitality that are the hallmarks of the ageless mind.

HISTORICAL PERSPECTIVE OF MINDFUL EATING

Tracing back through the annals of history, mindful eating is not a new concept, but an age-old practice embedded in various cultures. In ancient India, Ayurveda emphasized the importance of how and what we eat, considering it crucial for balance and health. Zen Buddhism introduced 'oryoki', a meditative form of eating that focuses on mindfulness and gratitude. Even the ancient Greeks had their symposiums, where food was a medium for philosophical discussions. Today, as we navigate a fast-paced, convenience-driven world, we revisit these ancient wisdoms to find balance in our eating habits.

THE SYMPHONY OF FOOD AND LIFE

Consider life as a grand orchestra, with each aspect contributing to a harmonious melody. In this orchestra, food plays a vital role, often underestimated, in the quality of the music we produce. It's not just sustenance; it's a source of pleasure, a medium for connection, and a way to nurture our body and soul. Through mindful eating, we learn to conduct this aspect of our lives with grace and awareness, allowing every meal to become an opportunity for mindfulness and joy.

MINDFUL EATING IN DIFFERENT CULTURES

Across the world, mindful eating manifests in various forms. In Japan, the traditional tea ceremony is not just about drinking tea but about mindfulness and aesthetics surrounding the act. Mediterranean cultures often focus on leisurely family meals, where food is a medium for connection and enjoyment. These diverse practices highlight a universal truth: the act of eating, when done mindfully, is a profound source of happiness and health.

As we delve deeper into this chapter, we will explore how mindful eating connects with our physical and mental well-being, offering practical tips to incorporate this practice into our daily lives. We'll explore its role in managing weight, enhancing digestion, and improving our mental state.

Alongside, we'll share stories like Emma's, who transformed her relationship with food through mindfulness, and discuss how mindful eating aligns with environmental consciousness and societal well-being.

By the end of this chapter, you will not only understand the art of mindful eating but also how to weave it into the fabric of your everyday life. It's a journey of rediscovery, connecting us with our food, our bodies, and our lives in profound ways.

THE CONNECTION BETWEEN MINDFUL EATING AND HEALTH

DIGESTIVE WELLNESS

The journey of mindful eating begins with its impact on our digestive wellness. When we eat mindfully, we slow down our eating process, chew our food thoroughly, and savor each bite. This not only enhances our enjoyment of the food but also significantly improves our digestion and nutrient absorption.

Scientific studies have shown that slower eating can lead to better digestion and even assist in managing gastrointestinal issues. For instance, a 2019 study published in the 'Journal of Gastroenterology and Hepatology' found that mindful eating practices could alleviate symptoms of irritable bowel syndrome.

WEIGHT MANAGEMENT

Mindful eating is not about strict diets or calorie counting; it's about developing a deeper understanding of our body's hunger and fullness cues. By paying attention to these signals, we can avoid overeating and make more nourishing food choices.

A 2020 research article in The American Journal of Clinical Nutrition highlighted how individuals practicing mindful eating were more likely to maintain a healthy weight, as it promotes eating in moderation and choosing quality foods over quantity.

HOLISTIC HEALTH BENEFITS

The benefits of mindful eating extend beyond physical health; they touch upon our mental and emotional well-being too. It encourages us to appreciate our meals, creating a sense of gratitude and satisfaction.

This approach can be particularly helpful in breaking the cycle of emotional eating, where we turn to food for comfort rather than hunger. By being present with our food, we learn to recognize these patterns and find healthier ways to cope with our emotions.

DEEPENING MINDFUL EATING PRACTICES

MINDFUL SHOPPING AND COOKING

Our journey with food begins long before we sit down to eat. It starts in the grocery store and continues in the kitchen. Mindful shopping involves choosing ingredients with attention and intention.

It's about being present during the selection process, considering the origin, nutritional value, and environmental impact of the food we buy. Emma, for instance, began to visit local farmers' markets, choosing fresh, locally sourced produce. She found that this not only supported her community but also made her feel more connected to her food.

Cooking, too, is an integral part of mindful eating. Engaging fully in the cooking process – from chopping vegetables to stirring a pot – can be a meditative and enjoyable experience. Emma discovered that by focusing on the process of cooking, she felt more relaxed and content. The act of preparing her meals became a joyful ritual rather than a chore.

SETTING THE SCENE FOR MINDFUL MEALS

Creating a conducive environment for eating is crucial for mindful dining. Emma made simple changes to her dining area to enhance her focus on meals.

She cleared the table of distractions, chose comfortable seating, and sometimes added elements like candles or soft music to create a calming atmosphere. These small adjustments made a significant difference in her dining experience, allowing her to be more present with her meals.

MINDFUL EATING WITH OTHERS

Sharing meals can be a communal and mindful experience. Emma learned to bring mindfulness into her social gatherings and family dinners. She encouraged conversations about the flavors, textures, and aromas of the food.

This not only enhanced the dining experience but also fostered deeper connections with her loved ones. Expressing gratitude collectively before meals became a cherished practice in her social circles.

THE PSYCHOLOGICAL ASPECTS OF MINDFUL EATING

UNDERSTANDING AND MANAGING EMOTIONAL EATING

One of the most transformative aspects of mindful eating for Emma was understanding her emotional relationship with food. Recognizing when she was eating in response to feelings rather than hunger was a breakthrough.

She learned to identify triggers for emotional eating and developed healthier coping mechanisms, such as going for a walk or practicing deep breathing.

MINDFULNESS IN FOOD CHOICES

Mindful eating also involves trusting our body's wisdom in making food choices. It's about developing a non-judgmental attitude towards ourselves and our eating habits.

Emma learned to listen to her body, choosing foods that nourished and satisfied her, rather than following rigid dietary rules. This shift in perspective brought a sense of peace and freedom in her relationship with food.

MINDFUL EATING IN SPECIAL SITUATIONS

The next section will explore how to maintain mindfulness in challenging eating environments, such as dining out, attending social events, and traveling. We will provide practical tips for making nourishing choices and staying connected with our eating experiences, even in less controlled settings.

EATING OUT MINDFULLY

Dining out is an integral part of our social lives, yet it often poses a challenge to mindful eating practices.

Emma found that with a few mindful strategies, she could still enjoy eating out without losing touch with her mindful eating habits.

- **MAKING NOURISHING CHOICES**
  Emma learned to scan menus for healthier options, focusing on dishes made with fresh, whole ingredients. She wasn't afraid to ask for modifications, like dressing on the side or extra vegetables.

- **PAYING ATTENTION TO PORTION SIZES**
  Restaurant servings are often larger than necessary. Emma adopted the habit of checking in with her hunger and fullness levels, eating slowly and mindfully. Sometimes, she would ask for half of her meal to be packed to take home.

- **EATING SLOWLY AND SAVORING EACH BITE**
  She reminded herself to eat slowly, putting down her cutlery between bites and engaging in conversation. This helped her enjoy the meal more fully and recognize satiety cues.

MINDFUL EATING AT SOCIAL EVENTS

Social events often revolve around food, which can make it easy to eat mindlessly. Emma used these gatherings as opportunities to practice and share her mindful eating habits.

- **FOCUSING ON SMALL SERVINGS**
  At buffets or potlucks, Emma would start with small servings, giving herself the chance to savor each item and decide if she truly wanted more.

- **ENGAGING IN MINDFUL CONVERSATION**

  Engaging in meaningful conversations during meals helped Emma stay present. She found that when she was mentally engaged, she was less likely to eat mindlessly.

- **PRACTICING GRATITUDE**

  At these events, Emma often led a moment of gratitude for the meal, sharing her practice with others and creating a mindful dining experience for everyone.

WHILE TRAVELING

Traveling presents its unique set of challenges for mindful eating, with new cuisines and changing routines. Emma developed strategies to maintain her practice even on the road.

- **PREPARING HEALTHY SNACKS**

  Knowing that healthy options might not always be available, Emma started packing nutritious snacks for her trips. This helped her avoid impulsive food choices when hunger struck unexpectedly.

- **RESEARCHING LOCAL FOODS**

  Part of Emma's travel preparation included researching local cuisines. She looked for healthy, authentic dining experiences, viewing them as an opportunity to expand her culinary horizons mindfully.

- **STAYING HYDRATED AND RESTED**

  Emma noticed that fatigue and dehydration often led to mindless eating. Keeping herself well-rested and hydrated became a priority, especially when adjusting to new time zones.

The Broader Impact of Mindful Eating

ENVIRONMENTAL AND SOCIETAL IMPLICATIONS

Mindful eating isn't just about our personal health; it has broader environmental and societal implications.

- **CONSCIOUS CONSUMERISM**
  Emma became more conscious of her food choices' environmental impact. She started choosing locally sourced, sustainable, and ethically produced food, reducing her carbon footprint and supporting local farmers.
- **COMMUNITY INVOLVEMENT**
  Sharing her mindful eating practices within her community, Emma started hosting workshops and dinner gatherings, spreading awareness about the benefits of this practice.

PERSONAL GROWTH

Mindful eating also became a gateway to broader personal growth for Emma.

- **GATEWAY TO BROADER MINDFULNESS**
  The principles of mindful eating spilled over into other areas of her life, leading to a more mindful approach to her work, relationships, and personal growth.

- **CULTIVATING PATIENCE AND COMPASSION**
  Through mindful eating, Emma developed greater patience and compassion, not just for herself but for others. She learned to approach life's challenges with a calm, centered mindset.

THE AGELESS BENEFITS OF MINDFUL EATING

As we explore the benefits of mindful eating, you'll discover how this practice can become a cornerstone of your youthful living journey. From weight management and digestive health to improved mental clarity and emotional well-being, the advantages are numerous.

BALANCED NUTRITION

Mindful eating encourages a balanced and varied diet, fostering overall health and vitality.

WEIGHT MANAGEMENT

By being attuned to hunger and fullness cues, we can naturally regulate our food intake, making it an effective tool for maintaining a healthy weight.

DIGESTIVE HARMONY

Mindful eating can alleviate digestive discomfort by promoting slower, more thorough chewing and enhancing the body's natural digestive processes.

STRESS REDUCTION

This practice fosters a sense of calm and reduces stress-related eating, contributing to mental and emotional well-being.

BRINGING MINDFUL EATING INTO YOUR LIFE

In this section, we'll delve into practical techniques and strategies for incorporating mindful eating into your daily routine. From mindful meal preparation to mindful snacking, you'll gain insights into how to infuse mindfulness into every aspect of your culinary journey.

CULTIVATING A MINDFUL RELATIONSHIP WITH FOOD

We'll explore the psychology of eating, including the role of emotional eating and ways to develop a healthier relationship with food. You'll learn how to discern between physical hunger and emotional cravings, enabling you to make choices that align with your well-being.

MINDFUL EATING AND BODY AWARENESS

Understanding the profound connection between mindful eating and body awareness is essential for cultivating a harmonious relationship with food and nourishing your ageless mind and body.

THE GIFT OF BODY AWARENESS

Body awareness is the practice of tuning in to the sensations and signals your body provides. It's about developing a deep understanding of your body's needs, cues, and responses. When combined with mindful eating, body awareness becomes a powerful tool for making conscious food choices.

One novel aspect of body awareness that we'll explore here is the concept of "mindful eating personas." Imagine that you have different personas or roles when it comes to eating. These personas represent your typical eating habits and patterns. By recognizing these personas, you gain insights into your relationship with food and can make changes.

- **THE SPEED RACER**
  This persona is always in a hurry when eating. Meals are consumed rapidly, often while multitasking or working. The Speed Racer rarely pauses to savor flavors or check in with hunger and fullness. To transform this persona, practice eating slowly, savoring each bite, and dedicating mealtime to eating only.

- **THE EMOTIONAL EATER**

    Emotional eating is a common challenge. This persona turns to food for comfort, stress relief, or to cope with emotions. Becoming aware of emotional triggers and finding alternative ways to address emotions, such as journaling or deep breathing, can help transform this persona.

- **THE MINDLESS MUNCHER**

    The Mindless Muncher often snacks absentmindedly, consuming calories without conscious awareness. To shift this persona, create designated snack times, and choose nutritious snacks. Avoid eating directly from a package to increase mindfulness.

- **THE GRAZER**

    Grazing throughout the day is the hallmark of this persona. Snacking occurs frequently, making it challenging to gauge hunger and fullness. Structuring regular mealtimes and incorporating mindful snack breaks can help bring balance to this persona.

- **THE CONSCIOUS CONSUMER**

    This persona embodies mindful eating principles. Meals are savored, and hunger and fullness cues are honored. The Conscious Consumer practices gratitude before meals and makes deliberate choices based on nutritional needs.

By recognizing your eating personas, you can identify patterns that may not align with mindful eating. This awareness enables you to consciously choose which persona to embody during meals and snacks, ultimately leading to a more mindful and balanced relationship with food.

THE HUNGER AND FULLNESS SCALE

One practical way to enhance body awareness during meals is by using the Hunger and Fullness Scale. This scale helps you recognize your body's hunger and fullness cues, allowing you to eat in alignment with your body's needs. It ranges from 1 (extremely hungry) to 10 (overly full). During meals, periodically pause to assess where you are on the scale. This practice can prevent overeating and promote a balanced intake of nourishment.

INTUITIVE EATING: TRUSTING YOUR BODY'S WISDOM

Intuitive eating is a holistic approach to nourishment that encourages you to trust your body's wisdom. It involves letting go of strict diets, calorie counting, and external food rules. Instead, you rely on internal cues like hunger, fullness, and cravings to guide your eating choices.

To practice intuitive eating, it's essential to reconnect with your body's signals. This includes differentiating between physical hunger and emotional hunger, as well as recognizing the sensations of satisfaction and fullness. Intuitive eating encourages you to eat when you're hungry and stop when you're satisfied, fostering a healthier and more intuitive relationship with food.

MINDFUL EATING AND BODY ACCEPTANCE

Body acceptance is a crucial aspect of body awareness and mindful eating. It involves embracing your body's unique shape and size without judgment or criticism. By practicing body acceptance, you cultivate a positive body image and reduce the tendency to engage in disordered eating behaviors.

Mindful eating can support body acceptance by encouraging you to focus on the nourishing aspects of food rather than its potential to change your body's appearance. When you eat mindfully, you're more likely to savor the flavors and textures of food, appreciate the nourishment it provides, and foster a sense of gratitude for your body's abilities.

MINDFUL EATING IN SOCIAL AND CULTURAL CONTEXTS

Eating is not just a solitary act; it's deeply woven into our social and cultural fabric. Understanding how to practice mindful eating in various social settings and cultural contexts is essential for maintaining mindfulness in real-life situations.

MINDFUL EATING WITH FAMILY AND FRIENDS

Eating with loved ones can be a joyful and social experience. However, it's common for mealtime conversations and distractions to take precedence over mindful eating. To practice mindful eating in social settings:

- Set an intention to be present during the meal.
- Engage in meaningful conversations without rushing.
- Savor each bite and enjoy the company of others.
- Encourage mindful eating as a shared experience.

NAVIGATING SOCIAL GATHERINGS

Social gatherings often involve abundant food options and the temptation to overindulge. To maintain mindfulness in such situations:

- Prioritize small, mindful portions of your favorite dishes.
- Choose nutrient-dense options when available.
- Focus on engaging with others rather than solely on the food.
- Listen to your body's hunger and fullness cues.

EXPLORING INTERNATIONAL CUISINES

When exploring international cuisines, embrace the opportunity to savor diverse flavors and cultural traditions. To practice mindful eating while trying new foods:

- Take time to appreciate the aromas and presentation of the dishes.
- Chew slowly and savor the unique flavors.
- Be open to new culinary experiences without judgment.
- Show respect for cultural customs and traditions.

CHALLENGES AND OPPORTUNITIES

Practicing mindful eating in social and cultural contexts may present challenges, but it also offers opportunities for growth and connection. Challenges may include peer pressure to overeat or distractions that hinder mindfulness. However, by applying the principles of mindful eating, you can navigate these challenges with grace and stay true to your mindful eating journey.

PRACTICAL TIPS: EMBRACING MINDFUL EATING

Now that we've explored the principles and benefits of mindful eating, let's delve into practical tips to help you embrace this transformative practice in your daily life.

These tips will guide you on your journey to cultivate a mindful relationship with food, nourishing not only your body but also your ageless mind.

BEGIN WITH GRATITUDE

Before every meal, take a moment to express gratitude for the food before you. Reflect on the effort that went into preparing the meal and the journey of the ingredients from the earth to your plate. This simple act of gratitude sets a mindful tone for your dining experience.

ENGAGE YOUR SENSES

As you sit down to eat, engage all your senses. Notice the colors, textures, and aromas of your food. Listen to the sounds of cooking or the quiet ambiance of your dining area. By involving all your senses, you create a fuller and more immersive experience.

MINDFUL MEAL PREPARATION

Extend mindfulness to the process of meal preparation. When selecting ingredients, appreciate their freshness and quality. As you chop vegetables or mix ingredients, immerse yourself in the act of cooking. Mindful meal preparation sets the stage for a mindful meal.

SET THE TABLE MINDFULLY

The way you set the table can influence your mindful eating experience. Arrange your plate, utensils, and glass with care. Use colors and textures that evoke a sense of calm and serenity. A well-set table can enhance the aesthetic pleasure of your meal.

MINDFUL BITES

During the meal, take small, mindful bites. Savor each morsel as if it were the first taste. Chew slowly and thoroughly, paying attention to the flavors and textures. Put your utensils down between bites to prevent mindless eating and to fully engage with your meal.

EAT WITH AWARENESS

As you eat, be fully present in the moment. Avoid distractions such as television, smartphones, or reading material. Focus solely on the act of eating and the sensations it brings. The more present you are, the more you'll enjoy and appreciate your food.

PAUSE BETWEEN BITES

One of the key principles of mindful eating is taking pauses between bites. After each bite, place your utensils down on your plate and take a moment of mindfulness. Close your eyes if you wish and tune in to the sensations in your body. These pauses allow your body to signal fullness, reducing the likelihood of overeating.

PORTION CONTROL

Pay attention to portion sizes. Use smaller plates and bowls to help control portion sizes and prevent overindulgence. Avoid eating directly from a large container, as it can lead to mindless eating. By controlling portions, you can maintain a healthy balance.

MINDFUL SNACKING

Extend mindful eating to snack times. Before reaching for a snack, pause for a moment of mindfulness. Ask yourself if you are truly hungry or if the desire to snack is driven by boredom, stress, or habit. Choose nutritious snacks and eat them mindfully, just as you would a meal.

HYDRATION AWARENESS

Remember that hydration is a vital aspect of mindful eating. Sip water mindfully throughout your meal to aid digestion and maintain hydration. Be attentive to your body's thirst cues and avoid excessive consumption of sugary or calorie-laden beverages.

CHEW THOROUGHLY

The act of chewing is fundamental to digestion. Chew your food thoroughly, breaking it down into smaller, more manageable pieces. Not only does this aid digestion, but it also allows you to fully savor the flavors.

EMOTIONAL AWARENESS

Develop emotional awareness around your eating habits. Before reaching for food, check in with your emotions. Are you genuinely hungry, or are you seeking food to cope with stress or emotions? Understanding your emotional triggers can lead to more conscious choices.

STRESS REDUCTION

Mindful eating can be a powerful tool for stress reduction. When stress tempts you to turn to food, pause for a moment of mindfulness. Take deep breaths to calm your nervous system. Ask yourself if you are truly hungry or if you are using food to soothe stress.

MINDFUL GROCERY SHOPPING

Extend mindfulness to your grocery shopping experience. Make a shopping list based on your nutritional goals and stick to it. Avoid impulsive purchases and processed foods. Choose fresh, whole ingredients with mindfulness and intention.

FOOD LABEL AWARENESS

When selecting packaged foods, be mindful of food labels. Read ingredient lists and nutrition facts with care. Choose foods that align with your nutritional goals and avoid products with excessive additives.

COOK WITH LOVE

Infuse your cooking process with love and intention. Approach cooking as a meditative practice, pouring positive energy into every dish. When you cook with love, your meals become nourishing on multiple levels.

MINDFUL EATING JOURNAL

Consider keeping a mindful eating journal. Record your experiences with mindful eating, including your observations, challenges, and moments of insight. Journaling can deepen your awareness and serve as a valuable reflection tool.

MINDFUL COOKING CLASSES

If you're interested in deepening your culinary skills and mindfulness, explore mindful cooking classes or workshops. These experiences can offer practical guidance and a supportive community of like-minded individuals.

By incorporating these practical tips into your daily life, you'll gradually cultivate the art of mindful eating. Remember that mindful eating is a journey, and each step you take brings you closer to a harmonious relationship with food and a more ageless mind and body.

Case Study 8:
A Journey Of Remarkable Change

To illustrate the transformative power of mindful eating, let me share with you the story of Jane, a woman who embarked on a journey to discover the profound impact of this practice on her life.

Jane had always been a busy professional, rushing from one meeting to another, grabbing fast food on the way, and barely taking a moment to breathe. She struggled with weight management and often felt stressed and fatigued. Her relationship with food was characterized by mindless eating and emotional binging.

One day, Jane stumbled upon a book on mindful eating. The concept intrigued her, and she decided to give it a try. She began with small steps, such as setting aside time to cook simple meals and eat without distractions. At first, it felt challenging. The urge to check her phone or multi-task was strong, but she persisted.

As Jane started practicing mindful eating, she noticed subtle changes. She savored the flavors of her meals, appreciating the effort she put into cooking. She took pauses between bites, allowing her body to signal fullness. Over time, she began to recognize the difference between physical hunger and emotional cravings.

One evening, Jane had a powerful breakthrough. She attended a dinner with friends, and instead of mindlessly devouring her food as she used to, she decided to fully engage in the practice of mindful eating. She tasted each bite as if it were the first time, appreciating the variety of flavors and textures on her plate. She engaged in meaningful conversations with her friends, sipping her water mindfully between bites. As the evening unfolded, Jane felt a deep sense of contentment and connection. She realized that food was not just about sustenance; it was about nourishing her body and soul. She discovered that mindful eating allowed her to savor life's moments more fully.

In the following months, Jane's journey continued. She lost weight gradually, not through restrictive diets but by listening to her body's cues and making conscious choices. Her stress levels decreased, and she found healthier ways to cope with her emotions, such as meditation and deep breathing exercises.

Jane's story is a testament to the transformative power of mindful eating. It's a practice that goes beyond the physical aspects of food; it's about nurturing a deeper connection with oneself and the world. Jane's ageless mind and vibrant spirit were a testament to the positive changes she experienced through mindful eating.

Conclusion For Chapter 8: Cultivating An Ageless Mind And Body

Throughout this chapter, we've seen how mindful eating much more than a dietary habit is — it's a holistic approach to life. By engaging in mindful eating, we don't just nourish our bodies; we also cultivate a sense of presence, gratitude, and connection.

This practice encourages us to slow down, savor each moment, and listen to our bodies, fostering a balanced relationship with food. As we have journeyed through the realms of mindful eating, we've uncovered practical tips and inspiring stories that demonstrate its transformative power.

As we conclude this chapter on mindful eating, it's essential to recapitulate the key points and insights gained from our exploration of this transformative practice.

Mindful eating, an art that intertwines the tranquility of meditation with the act of nourishment, offers a pathway to harmonize our physical and mental well-being, contributing significantly to the cultivation of an ageless mind and body.

Chapter Key Points

THE ESSENCE OF MINDFUL EATING

We started by understanding mindful eating as a practice that elevates our relationship with food from mere consumption to an act of mindfulness, echoing ancient traditions and contemporary needs.

CULTURAL PERSPECTIVES

We recognized that mindful eating is a global concept, valued in various cultures for its ability to enhance the dining experience and connect us more deeply with our meals.

HEALTH AND WELLNESS

Our discussion highlighted the health benefits of mindful eating, including improved digestion, weight management, and the alleviation of emotional eating patterns.

PRACTICAL IMPLEMENTATION

We delved into practical ways to incorporate mindful eating into daily life, from selecting and preparing food to creating the right environment for eating.

PSYCHOLOGICAL BENEFITS

We examined the psychological aspects of mindful eating, understanding how it helps manage emotional responses and encourages healthier eating choices.

MINDFUL EATING IN DIFFERENT SCENARIOS

The chapter also addressed how to maintain mindfulness in various challenging situations, such as eating out, attending social events, and traveling.

BROADER IMPACT

Finally, we explored the broader implications of mindful eating on environmental consciousness and personal growth.

SUMMARY AND PREPARATION FOR CHAPTER 9

In our last chapter, we will expand our exploration of holistic well-being. This upcoming chapter will delve into the transformative power of physical activity and its synergistic relationship with mindful eating. We will discover how exercise, much like mindful eating, is a cornerstone in our journey towards an ageless mind and body. This chapter will not only complement our understanding of mindful nutrition but also illuminate the role of physical activity in achieving a balanced and healthy lifestyle. Stay tuned for an invigorating exploration of how movement can be a powerful medicine for both the body and the mind, and how, when combined with mindful eating, it forms the foundation of a truly ageless existence.

Chapter 9
Movement As Medicine :
The Power Of Exercise

Introduction

Holistic well-being is like a tapestry, where every thread weaves together to form a beautiful picture of health and vitality. Physical exercise is a foundational and transformative thread that plays a crucial role in this tapestry.

In Chapter 9, we explore the significance of this thread and how it contributes to our overall well-being. We delve into the discipline of physical activity and discover how it complements and enhances the mental and emotional equilibrium that we strive for through meditation.

This chapter highlights the importance of incorporating regular exercise into our daily routine and how it can help us achieve a state of inner harmony and balance.

The Intersection Of Exercise And Meditation

At first glance, exercise and meditation might appear as distinct practices – one vigorous and dynamic, the other tranquil and still. However, the two are not just compatible; they are deeply interconnected. Meditation, as we have journeyed through in earlier chapters, brings clarity, peace, and balance to the mind and spirit. Exercise, on the other hand, is the yin to this yang, offering strength, vitality, and resilience to the body. Together, they form a holistic approach to well-being, each enhancing the benefits of the other.

In this chapter, we delve into how the physical rigor of exercise can lead to a meditative state of mind, where each movement syncs with breath, and awareness converges on the present moment.

This convergence is not just theoretical but is backed by science – studies have shown that regular physical activity significantly improves mental health, reduces stress and anxiety, and enhances cognitive function, all of which are also key benefits of meditation.

Why This Chapter Matters

"Why a chapter on exercise in a book about meditation?" one might ask. The answer lies in the holistic approach to health and wellness. True well-being is not achieved through focusing on one aspect of health in isolation. It's a multidimensional pursuit, where mental, emotional, and physical health are interlinked.

This chapter is a recognition of that truth, a guide to integrating exercise into your life in a way that supports and amplifies the benefits of your meditation practice.

What To Expect In This Chapter

UNDERSTANDING THE POWER OF PHYSICAL ACTIVITY

We begin by unraveling the science behind exercise and its extensive benefits. From improving cardiovascular health and muscle strength to enhancing brain function and mood, the role of exercise extends far beyond the gym.

TYPES OF EXERCISE FOR HOLISTIC HEALTH

Not all exercise is created equal. This section introduces various forms of exercise – cardiovascular, strength training, flexibility, balance exercises, and functional fitness – and explains how to select the right mix to suit your individual needs and goals.

THE MENTAL AND EMOTIONAL BENEFITS OF EXERCISE

Here, we explore the profound impact of physical activity on mental and emotional well-being. This connection highlights how exercise can be a potent tool in managing stress, combating anxiety and depression, and fostering a state of mindfulness.

CREATING A PERSONALIZED EXERCISE ROUTINE

Recognizing that every individual's journey and body are unique, this section provides practical guidance on how to create a personalized and sustainable exercise regimen.

INTEGRATING EXERCISE INTO DAILY LIFE

We offer creative and practical strategies to weave exercise into the fabric of your daily routine, making it an enjoyable and integral part of your life.

ADVANCED EXERCISE CONCEPTS

For those looking to deepen their fitness journey, this part of the chapter discusses advanced concepts like High-Intensity Interval Training (HIIT), the importance of rest and recovery, and injury prevention.

NUTRITION AND HYDRATION FOR OPTIMAL PERFORMANCE

Understanding that exercise is just part of the wellness equation, we delve into the role of nutrition and hydration, crucial for supporting an active lifestyle.

TRANSFORMATIONS THROUGH EXERCISE

Real-life stories of individuals who have transformed their lives through exercise not only serve as inspiration but also as tangible proof of the power of physical activity in enhancing life quality.

CONCLUSION

We tie everything together, emphasizing how exercise is a lifelong journey and its intrinsic connection to the practices of meditation and mindfulness.

AN INVITATION TO THE READER

As we embark on this exploration of exercise as a crucial component of holistic health, we invite you to approach this chapter not just as a guide to physical fitness but as a journey towards a more balanced, healthier, and fulfilled life.

The stories, strategies, and insights presented here aim to inspire, inform, and empower you to embrace exercise as a natural ally in your quest for well-being.

Whether you are a seasoned athlete or someone who's more familiar with the comfort of a couch than the sweat of a workout, this chapter has something for you. It's designed to be inclusive, practical, and motivational, offering pathways to incorporate exercise into your life, regardless of your current fitness level or lifestyle.

In reading this chapter, we hope you find not only the motivation to move and strengthen your body but also to discover the profound and often overlooked connection between physical activity and the serene world of meditation. Let this be the chapter that bridges the gap between motion and stillness, between strength and serenity, guiding you towards a life where body and mind coexist in harmonious balance.

THE PHYSIOLOGICAL BENEFITS OF REGULAR EXERCISE

HEART HEALTH

Exercise strengthens the heart, improving its efficiency in pumping blood throughout the body. Regular physical activity reduces the risk of heart diseases by lowering blood pressure, improving cholesterol levels, and enhancing overall cardiovascular health.

DIABETES MANAGEMENT AND PREVENTION

Regular exercise helps in regulating blood sugar levels and increases insulin sensitivity, which can prevent or manage type 2 diabetes.

WEIGHT MANAGEMENT

While diet plays a critical role in weight management, exercise is essential in maintaining healthy body weight. It helps in burning calories, building muscle, and boosting metabolism.

BONE DENSITY AND MUSCLE STRENGTH

Weight-bearing exercises, such as walking, running, and resistance training, strengthen bones and muscles, reducing the risk of osteoporosis and sarcopenia (muscle loss) as we age.

IMMUNE SYSTEM BOOST

Moderate intensity exercise can boost the immune system by promoting good circulation, which allows cells and substances of the immune system to move through the body freely and do their job efficiently.

MENTAL AND EMOTIONAL BENEFITS OF EXERCISE

STRESS RELIEF

Physical activity increases concentrations of norepinephrine, a chemical that moderates the brain's response to stress. Regular exercise also reduces levels of the body's stress hormones, such as adrenaline and cortisol.

MOOD ENHANCEMENT

Exercise stimulates the release of endorphins, often known as 'feel-good hormones', which create feelings of happiness and euphoria. This is why exercise is often recommended for people battling depression and anxiety.

IMPROVED SLEEP

Regular physical activity can help you fall asleep faster, sleep more deeply, and wake feeling more energetic and refreshed.

BOOST IN SELF-CONFIDENCE

Achieving exercise goals, whether big or small, can boost self-esteem and body image.

COGNITIVE HEALTH

Exercise improves brain function in both direct and indirect ways. It directly affects the brain by reducing insulin resistance, reducing inflammation, and stimulating the release of growth factors—chemicals in the brain that affect the health of brain cells.

DEBUNKING COMMON EXERCISE MYTHS

As we recognize the extensive benefits of exercise, it's important to address and debunk common myths that might hinder someone's willingness to engage in regular physical activity:

Myth: Exercise needs to be intense and prolonged to be effective.

Truth: Even moderate-intensity activities, like brisk walking or gardening, can have significant health benefits.

Myth: I'm too old to start exercising.

Truth: It's never too late to start. Even moderate physical activity can improve the health of people who are frail or have diseases associated with aging.

Myth: Exercise will make me tired.

Truth: Regular exercise actually boosts energy levels and helps in improving overall physical stamina.

Myth: I need to go to the gym to get a good workout.

Truth: Effective workouts can be done anywhere – at home, in a park, or even in a small space with minimal or no equipment.

In summary, the power of physical activity extends far beyond mere physical appearance or fitness. It encompasses a vast array of benefits that cater to our physical, mental, and emotional well-being. In the following sections, we'll explore the various forms of exercise and how to integrate them into your daily life for holistic health.

TYPES OF EXERCISE FOR HOLISTIC HEALTH

1. CARDIOVASCULAR EXERCISE

Definition and Examples: Cardiovascular or aerobic exercises are activities that raise your heart rate and breathing. They include running, swimming, cycling, brisk walking, rowing, and even dancing.

Heart Health: Cardio exercises strengthen the heart muscle, improving its pumping efficiency and reducing the resting heart rate. This can lower the risk of heart disease and stroke.

Endurance and Stamina: Regular cardio boosts lung capacity and endurance, making daily activities easier and less fatiguing.

Weight Management: These exercises are effective in burning calories and are a key component of any weight loss or weight management plan.

Mental Health Benefits: Cardio activities have a significant impact on reducing symptoms of depression and anxiety. They release endorphins, natural mood lifters, enhancing a sense of well-being.

Sleep and Energy Levels: Engaging in regular cardiovascular exercise can improve sleep quality and elevate energy levels all day long

2. STRENGTH TRAINING

Understanding Strength Training: This form of exercise involves the use of resistance to induce muscular contraction, which builds the strength, anaerobic endurance, and size of skeletal muscles.

Types of Strength Training: It includes using free weights, weight machines, resistance bands, or bodyweight exercises like push-ups and squats.

Benefits for Aging: As we age, we lose muscle mass and strength. Strength training can counteract this decline, maintaining muscle tone and bone density.

Metabolic Benefits: These exercises enhance metabolic rate, which is crucial for weight management and controlling blood sugar levels.

Mental Health: Strength training has been linked to improved cognitive function, reduced anxiety and depression symptoms, and enhanced self-esteem.

3. FLEXIBILITY EXERCISES

The Role of Flexibility: Flexibility exercises enhance the ability of your muscles and joints to move through their full range of motion. They are crucial in preventing injuries and can reduce pain and stiffness.

Yoga and Pilates: Yoga combines physical postures, breathing exercises, meditation, and a distinct philosophy. Pilates focuses on strengthening the body, often with an emphasis on the core.

Stretching: Traditional stretching exercises are simple yet effective in improving flexibility, posture, and can be a great way to relax and release tension.

Mental and Emotional Benefits: Practices like yoga and Pilates offer a meditative component, reducing stress, and promoting mental clarity and inner peace.

4. BALANCE EXERCISES

Importance of Balance Training: Balance exercises are crucial, especially as we age, for preventing falls, which can lead to serious injuries.

Activities for Balance: They include standing on one foot, heel-to-toe walk, tai chi, and certain yoga poses like the tree pose.

Cognitive Benefits: Balance exercises are not just physical; they also challenge your brain and can improve cognitive function.

5. FUNCTIONAL FITNESS

Real-World Exercise: Functional fitness exercises are designed to train and develop your muscles to make it easier and safer to perform everyday activities, such as carrying groceries or playing a game of basketball with your kids.

Examples of Functional Exercises: These include multi-directional lunges, stair climbing, and exercises that mimic lifting, squatting, and reaching.

Benefits for Daily Life: These exercises improve balance, agility, and muscle strength, reducing the risk of injury in daily activities.

6. COMBINING DIFFERENT TYPES FOR HOLISTIC BENEFITS

Creating a Balanced Workout Routine: For optimal health benefits, a combination of different types of exercise is recommended. This might include cardio exercises for heart health, strength training for muscle maintenance, flexibility exercises for joint health, and balance training for stability.

Individual Tailoring: Everyone's needs and abilities are different. It's important to tailor your exercise routine to your personal goals, fitness level, and any health conditions you might have.

OVERCOMING BARRIERS TO EXERCISE

TIME MANAGEMENT

One of the biggest barriers to regular exercise is a lack of time. Incorporating short bursts of activity throughout the day or choosing exercises that provide multiple benefits (like swimming or yoga) can be effective strategies.

MOTIVATION

Staying motivated can be challenging. Setting realistic goals, tracking progress, and engaging in activities you enjoy can help maintain regular exercise habits.

ACCESSIBILITY

Not everyone has access to a gym or expensive equipment. However, many effective exercises can be done at home with minimal or no equipment.

Safety And Injury Prevention

WARM-UP AND COOL-DOWN

It's essential to warm up before exercising and cool down afterward to prevent injuries.

LISTENING TO YOUR BODY

Paying attention to what your body tells you during and after exercise can help avoid overtraining and injury.

PROFESSIONAL GUIDANCE

Especially for beginners or those with specific health conditions, seeking guidance from fitness professionals can be beneficial.

Exercise And The Brain: A Mental Boost

1. COGNITIVE FUNCTION AND BRAIN HEALTH

Neurological Impact of Exercise: Regular physical activity has a direct, positive effect on brain structure and function. It increases the flow of blood, oxygen, and nutrients to the brain, enhancing overall cognitive abilities.

Neurogenesis and Neuroplasticity: Exercise stimulates the production of neurotrophic factors, which support the growth and survival of neurons. This leads to neurogenesis (growth of new brain cells) and neuroplasticity (the brain's ability to adapt and change).

Memory and Concentration: Aerobic exercises, in particular, have been shown to increase the size of the hippocampus, the brain area involved in verbal memory and learning.

Cognitive Decline Prevention: Regular physical activity is linked with a lower risk of cognitive decline and dementia in older adults.

2. STRESS REDUCTION

Physiological Response to Exercise: Exercise reduces levels of the body's stress hormones, such as adrenaline and cortisol. It also stimulates the production of endorphins, the body's natural painkillers and mood elevators.

The Role of Endorphins: These chemicals produced in the brain during exercise can lead to feelings of euphoria, often referred to as the "runner's high."

Managing Chronic Stress: Regular exercise can help in the management of chronic stress, promoting a more balanced mental state.

3. ENHANCED CREATIVITY AND MENTAL CLARITY

Boosting Brain Power: Physical activity can clear the mind and help you think more creatively. After a workout, the brain's functionality improves, leading to clearer thinking and better problem-solving abilities.

The Mind-Body Connection: Engaging in exercise can also be a form of moving meditation, improving focus and mental clarity.

Creative Thinking: Studies suggest that walking, in particular, can boost creative ideation in real-time and shortly after.

4. COMBATTING ANXIETY AND DEPRESSION

Mental Health Benefits: Exercise is a powerful depression fighter. It promotes neural growth, reduces inflammation, and creates a calming effect on the brain.

Anxiety Reduction: Regular participation in aerobic exercise has been shown to decrease overall levels of tension, elevate and stabilize mood, improve sleep, and improve self-esteem.

The Role of Regular Exercise: Even five minutes of aerobic exercise can stimulate anti-anxiety effects, making it a powerful tool for managing mental health.

5. MINDFULNESS AND EXERCISE

Exercise as a Mindful Practice: Certain forms of exercise, like yoga, tai chi, and Pilates, are inherently mindful, requiring concentration and focus on the present moment, which can lead to improved mental and emotional states.

Mindful Running/Walking: This involves focusing on the physical sensation of walking or running, such as the rhythm of your breathing, the feeling of your feet touching the ground, and the wind against your face.

The Benefits of Mindful Movement: This practice can improve mental focus, reduce symptoms of stress and anxiety, and contribute to a deeper sense of peace and well-being.

6. ENHANCING SLEEP QUALITY

Impact on Sleep Patterns: Exercise can contribute to more sound and restful sleep. Regular physical activity can help you fall asleep faster and deepen your sleep, leaving you feeling more rested.

The Timing of Exercise: Timing can be key, as exercising too close to bedtime may leave you too energized to fall asleep.

7. BUILDING RESILIENCE

Developing Mental Fortitude: Regular exercise can help you build resilience and cope in a healthy way with life's challenges. The discipline and dedication required for consistent exercise can foster a sense of purpose and resilience.

Stress and Adversity Management: Physical activity can be a healthy outlet for relieving stress and processing emotions, contributing to greater resilience in facing life's ups and downs.

8. EXERCISE AND AGING

Maintaining Cognitive Function in Aging: Regular physical activity is particularly important in older adults as it can help boost cognitive functions that tend to decline with age.

Social Aspects of Exercise in Aging: Group exercises or fitness classes can also provide social benefits, reducing feelings of loneliness and isolation among older adults.

9. PRACTICAL TIPS FOR INCORPORATING EXERCISE FOR MENTAL HEALTH

Finding Activities You Enjoy: Choose activities that you enjoy and look forward to doing. Enjoyment is key to maintaining consistency in any exercise routine.

Setting Realistic Goals: Set achievable goals to stay motivated. Track your progress to see how far you've come.

Incorporating Variety: Keep your routine interesting by trying different types of exercises. This not only keeps you engaged but also ensures all-around fitness.

In summary, the impact of exercise on the brain and mental health is profound and multi-faceted. From enhancing cognitive functions and reducing stress to fostering resilience and improving sleep, physical activity is an invaluable component of mental and emotional well-being. In the following sections, we will explore how to create a personalized exercise routine that aligns with your lifestyle and how to integrate these exercises into your daily life for optimal mental, emotional, and physical health.

Creating A Personalized Exercise Routine

Creating an exercise routine that is tailored to your individual needs, preferences, and lifestyle is crucial for maintaining consistency and achieving your health goals. This section provides guidance on how to create a personalized exercise plan.

1. ASSESSING YOUR FITNESS LEVEL

Initial Assessment: Before starting any exercise program, it's important to assess your current fitness level. This might include considering factors like your cardiovascular endurance, strength, flexibility, and balance.

Health Check: If you have any health concerns or are new to regular exercise, it's advisable to consult with a healthcare provider or a fitness professional.

2. SETTING REALISTIC GOALS

Short-term and Long-term Goals: Set achievable short-term goals that lead to larger, long-term objectives. Goals should be Specific, Measurable, Achievable, Relevant, and Time-bound (SMART).

Examples of Goals: This could be anything from walking 30 minutes a day, five days a week, to completing a 5K run in three months.

3. DEVELOPING A BALANCED WORKOUT PLAN

Incorporating Different Types of Exercise: A well-rounded exercise routine includes a mix of cardiovascular, strength, flexibility, and balance exercises.

Applying the FITT Principle: To structure your workout, consider the Frequency, Intensity, Time, and Type (FITT) of exercise. This helps in creating a balanced and varied exercise program.

4. OVERCOMING BARRIERS TO EXERCISE

Time Management: For those with busy schedules, it might involve short but intense workouts, or integrating physical activity into daily routines, like cycling to work or taking the stairs.

Lack of Motivation: Staying motivated can be challenging. Try to find an exercise buddy, join a class, or use fitness apps that track and reward progress.

5. BUILDING A ROUTINE

Start Slowly: If you are new to exercise or returning after a break, start with low-intensity activities and gradually increase the intensity.

Consistency is Key: Aim for consistency rather than intensity at the beginning. Even short 10-15 minute sessions can be effective.

6. ADAPTING THE ROUTINE TO LIFE CHANGES

Flexible Approach: Life circumstances change, and your exercise routine should be adaptable. This could mean switching to different types of exercise during busy periods or as you age.

Listening to Your Body: Pay attention to how your body responds to exercise and be willing to adjust your routine accordingly.

7. TRACKING YOUR PROGRESS

Monitoring Your Activities: Keeping a log of your workouts and noting how you feel can be motivating and informative. It helps in tracking progress and identifying patterns.

Adjustments Based on Feedback: Use the feedback from your body and your progress logs to make necessary adjustments to your routine.

8. SAFETY FIRST

Warming Up and Cooling Down: Include a warm-up and a cool-down in your routine to prevent injuries. A warm-up could include light cardio and dynamic stretches. Cooling down might involve slower movements and static stretching.

Proper Technique: Ensure you are using the correct form, especially when lifting weights or doing complex movements. Incorrect technique can lead to injuries.

9. INCORPORATING FUN AND ENJOYMENT

Choose Activities You Enjoy: The more you enjoy your exercise routine, the more likely you are to stick with it. This could be dancing classes, outdoor hiking, or team sports.

Trying New Things: Keep things interesting by trying new activities or mixing up your routine.

YOGA AND PILATES: MIND-BODY EXERCISE

In this section, we delve into the realms of yoga and Pilates, exploring their unique contributions as mind-body exercises that blend physical activity with mental and emotional wellness.

1. YOGA: A HOLISTIC PRACTICE

Origins and Philosophy: Yoga, with its origins in ancient India, is more than physical exercise; it's a holistic practice that integrates physical postures (asanas), breath control (pranayama), and meditation (dhyana). We explore the philosophy and various styles of yoga, each offering a unique approach to wellness.

Benefits Beyond Flexibility: While yoga is renowned for enhancing flexibility, its benefits extend to stress reduction, improved mental clarity, and emotional balance. Regular practice can lead to improved balance, digestive health, and even bolster the immune system.

2. PILATES: STRENGTH AND ALIGNMENT

The Pilates Method: Developed by Joseph Pilates, this form of exercise emphasizes controlled movements, core strength, and mindful breathing. We discuss how Pilates balances muscle development with flexibility and mental concentration.

Adaptable for All Ages: Pilates is suitable for all fitness levels and ages. It's particularly effective in improving posture, muscle tone, and alignment. We highlight how Pilates can be adapted for different bodies and needs, making it an excellent choice for injury prevention and overall body awareness.

3. THE MIND-BODY CONNECTION

Integration with Meditation: Both yoga and Pilates offer meditative components that align closely with the principles of meditation discussed in earlier chapters. This section elaborates on how these practices enhance body awareness, anchor the mind in the present moment, and cultivate a sense of inner peace.

INTEGRATING EXERCISE INTO DAILY LIFE

Incorporating exercise into your daily routine is essential for sustained physical activity and achieving holistic health. This section offers practical tips and strategies for making exercise a natural and enjoyable part of your everyday life.

1. MAKING EXERCISE A HABIT

Routine Integration: Aim to make exercise a non-negotiable part of your daily routine, much like eating or sleeping. Schedule it as a regular activity in your day.

Cue-Based Habits: Associate exercise with specific cues or triggers in your day. For example, a morning workout could follow your first cup of coffee.

2. UTILIZING ACTIVE COMMUTING

Active Travel Choices: If possible, choose walking or cycling over driving or public transport for short trips. This not only incorporates physical activity into your day but also contributes to environmental well-being.

Benefits of Active Commuting: Active commuting has been shown to improve mental well-being, reduce stress, and increase daily physical activity levels.

3. WORKPLACE WELLNESS

Desk Exercises: Incorporate simple exercises you can do at your desk, like seated leg lifts or desk push-ups.

Movement Breaks: Take short, regular breaks to stand, stretch, or walk. Use a standing desk if available.

4. EXERCISE WITH FAMILY OR FRIENDS

Group Activities: Engage in physical activities with family or friends. This not only makes exercising more enjoyable but also helps in building a support system.

Weekend Activities: Plan active weekends, like hiking, biking, or playing a sport together.

5. INCORPORATING PHYSICAL ACTIVITY INTO HOUSEHOLD CHORES

Active Chores: Turn household chores into opportunities for exercise. Activities like gardening, vacuuming, or washing the car can be good physical workouts.

6. SHORT, HIGH-INTENSITY WORKOUTS

Efficient Exercise: For those pressed for time, high-intensity interval training (HIIT) offers an efficient way to exercise. These are short bursts of intense activity followed by brief rest periods.

HIIT Benefits: HIIT workouts can be done in as little as 15-20 minutes and have been shown to improve cardiovascular health, strength, and metabolic rate.

7. LEVERAGING TECHNOLOGY

Fitness Apps and Online Resources: Use technology to your advantage. Fitness apps can track your activity, provide workout ideas, and even offer virtual coaching.

Online Classes: With the proliferation of online fitness classes, you have access to a variety of workouts from the comfort of your home.

8. MINDFUL MOVEMENT

Integrating Mindfulness: Practice mindfulness during exercise by focusing on your body's movements and how it feels, rather than just going through the motions.

Yoga and Tai Chi: Activities like yoga and tai chi are excellent for combining physical movement with mindfulness, enhancing both mental and physical health.

9. ADAPTING TO CHANGING CIRCUMSTANCES

Flexible Approaches: Be adaptable with your exercise routine. Life changes, and so should your approach to physical activity. This could mean trying different types of exercise or adjusting the intensity and duration of your workouts.

10. STAYING MOTIVATED

Tracking Progress: Keep track of your physical activity and celebrate your achievements, no matter how small. This can be a powerful motivator.

Variety in Exercise: Keep your routine interesting by regularly trying new activities or changing your workout regimen.

11. MAKING EXERCISE ENJOYABLE

Fun Factor: Choose activities that you genuinely enjoy. If you like what you are doing, you are more likely to stick with it.

Music and Entertainment: Listening to music, podcasts, or audiobooks during exercise can make it more enjoyable.

12. SETTING REALISTIC EXPECTATIONS

Patience and Consistency: Understand that progress takes time. Set realistic expectations and be patient with yourself as you build up your fitness.

By integrating these strategies into your daily life, exercise becomes less of a chore and more of a natural and enjoyable part of your routine. In the next sections, we will delve into specific types of exercises such as Yoga and Pilates and explore their unique benefits for holistic health.

IMPORTANCE OF REST AND RECOVERY

RECOVERY

Adequate rest is crucial for muscle repair, strength building, and performance improvement. Overtraining can lead to injuries and burnout.

ACTIVE RECOVERY

Incorporating light exercise like walking or gentle yoga on rest days can aid in recovery and mobility.

INJURY PREVENTION

Technique and Form: Proper technique is essential to prevent injuries, especially in weightlifting and complex movements.

Listening to Your Body: Paying attention to your body's signals and not pushing through pain is important for long-term fitness.

NUTRITION AND HYDRATION FOR OPTIMAL PERFORMANCE

Effective exercise goes hand-in-hand with proper nutrition and hydration.

NUTRITIONAL NEEDS

Balanced Diet: A balanced diet rich in carbohydrates, proteins, healthy fats, vitamins, and minerals is essential for energy and recovery.

PRE- AND POST-WORKOUT NUTRITION

Consuming the right nutrients before and after exercise can improve performance and speed up recovery.

HYDRATION

Staying Hydrated: Adequate hydration is crucial for optimal physical performance. Water regulates body temperature, lubricates joints, and helps transport nutrients for energy.

Hydration Guidelines: Drink water before, during, and after exercise. The amount depends on the intensity of the workout and individual needs.

Metamorphosis Through Exercise: Unveiling Your Potential

In this section, we explore heartfelt stories of individuals whose lives were profoundly transformed through exercise. These narratives offer a glimpse into the real-world impact of physical activity, resonating with challenges, triumphs, and the profound connection between body and mind.

1. Emily's Escape: From Anxiety to Marathon Runner

Backstory: Emily, a 35-year-old graphic designer, battled anxiety for years. Juggling work and family life, she often felt overwhelmed, leading to sleepless nights and constant fatigue.

A Chance Encounter: Her journey began unexpectedly when she joined a colleague for a casual evening jog. Initially reluctant, she found surprising solace in the rhythmic motion of running.

The Transformation: Over months, Emily's casual jogs turned into a passion. Running became her therapy, her time to unwind and reflect. She built up her stamina, and to her own astonishment, completed her first marathon. The physical achievement was impressive, but more so was her mental transformation. Running taught her resilience, helped manage her anxiety, and brought a newfound confidence that transcended into all aspects of her life.

2. DAVID'S COMEBACK: REBUILDING AFTER INJURY

Backstory: A former semi-professional soccer player, David's world turned upside down following a severe knee injury. The injury not only halted his career but plunged him into a state of depression.

The Road to Recovery: His path to recovery began in a rehabilitation center where he discovered the gentle art of Pilates. Pilates, with its focus on controlled movements and core strength, became his gateway back to fitness.

Rediscovering Himself: As his strength returned, so did his spirit. David found joy in coaching young soccer players, sharing his love for the sport in a new way. His journey through injury and recovery reshaped his perspective on life, teaching him the value of patience and the power of adaptability.

3. ANITA'S VICTORY OVER AGE: A SENIOR'S JOURNEY TO EMPOWERMENT

Backstory: At 67, Anita felt the encroaching limitations of age. A retired school teacher, she longed to be active in her golden years but was hindered by joint pains and a fear of injury. Encouraged by friends, she hesitantly joined a senior yoga class. What started as a tentative step soon blossomed into a journey of self-discovery.

Renewed Vigor: Yoga brought more than physical flexibility; it revived her spirit. Anita's mornings were now filled with sun salutations, her days with newfound energy. She became an inspiration in her community, leading wellness initiatives for fellow seniors. Her story is a testament to the fact that it's never too late to start and that age is just a number when it comes to embracing life.

CONCLUSION FOR CHAPTER 9: THE SYNERGY OF EXERCISE AND MEDITATION FOR HOLISTIC WELL-BEING

As we reach the culmination of our journey in this final chapter, we are reminded of the profound synergy between exercise and meditation, and their transformative impact on holistic well-being. Through the stories of Emily, David, and Anita, we've witnessed how these practices extend far beyond physical health, touching the very essence of our mental and emotional lives.

This chapter serves as a powerful testament to the idea that exercise is not a mere physical routine but a bridge to a harmonious existence, nourishing every facet of our being. Emily's shift from anxiety to serenity,

David's transformation from stress to resilience, and Anita's journey from fatigue to vitality vividly illustrate how exercise and meditation can elevate our mental and emotional states.

As we embark on the final leg of our ageless living journey, let us carry with us the profound understanding that well-being is not an endpoint but a continuous, ever-evolving path.

It's the realization that exercise and meditation are not separate entities but interconnected elements of a rich, fulfilling life.

In the chapters we leave behind, and in those that await us in the future, we continue to explore ageless living, empowered by the knowledge that by harmonizing body and mind, we unlock the door to a life characterized by boundless vitality, enduring youth, and profound well-being.

Chapter Key Points

DIVERSE EXERCISE FORMS

We explored various exercises, from cardiovascular to strength training, each offering unique benefits for physical and mental health.

EXERCISE'S MENTAL AND EMOTIONAL IMPACT:

The significant role of physical activity in reducing stress, enhancing mood, and improving cognitive function was emphasized.

CUSTOMIZING EXERCISE PLANS

Strategies to create personalized exercise routines that align with individual needs and goals were discussed.

INTEGRATING EXERCISE INTO DAILY LIFE

Practical tips for making exercise a seamless part of daily routines were provided.

ADVANCED FITNESS CONCEPTS

The chapter delved into HIIT, the importance of rest, and injury prevention, catering to those seeking to deepen their fitness journey.

NUTRITIONAL AND HYDRATION SUPPORT

The role of a balanced diet and adequate hydration in complementing an active lifestyle was highlighted.

INSPIRATIONAL STORIES

Real-life stories showcased the life-changing impact of regular exercise on individuals from various walks of life.

FINAL REFLECTIONS
The Essence of Our Journey

As we reach the culmination of this book, it is time to pause and reflect on the profound journey we have undertaken together. From the initial steps into the serene world of meditation in Chapter 1, to the dynamic realms of physical exercise in Chapter 9, our exploration has spanned far beyond the boundaries of traditional mindfulness practices.

This journey has been a tapestry woven with threads of self-discovery, balance, and enriched living, each chapter adding its unique hue and texture to the overall picture of holistic well-being.

The TakeAway:
Meditation As A Lifelong Companion

Meditation, as revealed through the pages of this book, emerges not merely as a practice but as a lifelong companion. This journey, sprinkled with insights and techniques, unveils meditation as a multifaceted tool - a beacon guiding us through the fog of mental clutter, a stabilizer balancing our emotional tides, and a whispering ally in our quest for physical harmony.

Each chapter has unfolded layers of this journey, revealing how meditation intertwines with every aspect of our existence, from stress reduction and emotional well-being to cognitive enhancement and physical vitality.

Applying The Lessons Learned

As you step forward from here, carry the essence of these teachings within you. Let the flexibility and adaptability of meditation mold seamlessly into the contours of your life. Whether it's integrating mindfulness into a morning routine, as suggested in Chapter 7, or embracing the meditative rhythm of a run, as explored in Chapter 9, these practices are designed to fluidly become part of your everyday existence. The key lies in consistency, a willingness to adapt, and an openness to the ever-evolving journey of self-growth.

The "So What" Factor

What does this journey mean for you? It signifies empowerment - the realization that the keys to a transformative life lie within your grasp. Through meditation and its allied practices, you possess the ability to not just weather the storms of life but to dance in the rain. This journey is about more than finding tranquility in silence; it's about infusing that tranquility into the cacophony of daily life, turning every moment into an opportunity for growth, insight, and joy.

A Compelling Future

Envision a future where challenges are met with equanimity, where each day is imbued with a deep sense of presence, and where your interactions are rich and profound. This is the future that meditation promises - a life where stillness and action, contemplation and engagement, peace and vitality coexist in beautiful harmony. It's a future where meditation is not an escape from reality but a deeper engagement with it.

Your Journey Awaits

As this book draws to a close, remember that your journey is just beginning. Each new day presents a canvas to practice mindfulness, to grow, and to live with intention. Meditation, as we have discovered, is not a static destination but a dynamic path - a path that meanders through the landscapes of your inner world, uncovering hidden treasures of wisdom, strength, and serenity.

Your journey forward is one of endless discovery, a voyage towards an ageless life marked by balance, mindfulness, and an ever-deepening understanding of yourself and the world around you. Embrace this journey with enthusiasm and curiosity. Let meditation, along with its companions of mindful eating and physical exercise, be your guides in this adventure of a lifetime.

Here's to your journey, one that transcends the pages of this book and weaves into the fabric of your daily life. A journey not just to a destination of peace and balance but through a life lived fully, mindfully, and richly. Your path to ageless living awaits – a path adorned with discovery, growth, and boundless potential.

REFERENCES

NOTE TO READERS:

In *The Ageless Mind,* I explore the transformative world of meditation and its influence on aging and stress management. This book is a blend of my personal experiences, enriched by a decade of Transcendental Meditation practice, and insights from various cultural perspectives.

While a formal list of references is not included, the book is informed by a range of sources that reflect the depth and diversity of meditation practice. On the final page are some general references that have influenced some of the writing and thinking in this book, offering readers a starting point for their exploration.

GENERAL REFERENCES:

Kabat-Zinn, J. (1994). "Wherever You Go, There You Are: Mindfulness Meditation in Everyday Life."

Nhat Hanh, T. (1999). "The Miracle of Mindfulness: An Introduction to the Practice of Meditation."

Davidson, R.J., & Begley, S. (2012). "The Emotional Life of Your Brain."

Goleman, D., & Davidson, R.J. (2017). "Altered Traits: Science Reveals How Meditation Changes Your Mind, Brain, and Body."

Wallace, B.A. (2006). "The Attention Revolution: Unlocking the Power of the Focused Mind."

Harris, S. (2014). "Waking Up: A Guide to Spirituality Without

Religion."

Benson, H. (2000). "The Relaxation Response."

Siegel, D.J. (2007). "The Mindful Brain: Reflection and Attunement in the Cultivation of Well-Being."

Rosenthal, N.E. (2012). "Transcendence: Healing and Transformation Through Transcendental Meditation."

Lutz, A., Slagter, H.A., Dunne, J.D., & Davidson, R.J. (2008). "Attention

Ambrose Hines

www.ingramcontent.com/pod-product-compliance
Lightning Source LLC
Chambersburg PA
CBHW070152100426
42743CB00013B/2891